VITAMIN E

Vitamin E h r it is
an invaluab tion
against such ease
and skin con w to
get the best the
optimum inta t.

VITAMIN E:
The Vitality Vitamin

by

DR LEONARD MERVYN

NATURE'S WAY

THORSONS PUBLISHERS LIMITED
Wellingborough, Northamptonshire

First published 1980
Second Impression 1981

ISBN 0 7225 0533 7

Photoset by
Specialised Offset Services Limited, Liverpool.
Reproduced, printed and bound in Great Britain by
Cox & Wyman Ltd., Reading.

CONTENTS

INTRODUCTION

Amongst all the vitamins, there is none more calculated to cause controversy in the medical profession than vitamin E when it comes to claims concerning its usefulness in man. At various times it has been claimed to help in heart disease, blood circulation disorders, reproductive problems, diseases of the nervous system and in skin injuries, including burns.

The vitamin is also alleged to prevent ageing, to protect against the effects of air pollution and, on a more popular note, to help performance in the athletic and the sexual fields.

While such a wide variety of claims has been used by its critics as good reason why vitamin E is not the wonder vitamin it appears to be, it is not unusual for the medical profession to accept other 'wonder' drugs.

During the 1940's, penicillin was recognized as the cure-all antibiotic, yet its abuse by the medical profession led to an ever decreasing effectiveness.

The 'wonder' drugs of the 1950's were the corticosteroids, of which the forerunner was the naturally-occurring hydrocortisone. These steroids were used to treat just about every degenerative disease and allergic condition diagnosed, yet they turned out to be effective in only a limited number of cases. They produced side-effects that were often worse than the condition being treated.

Came the 1960's and the great surge was in the drugs known as Beta-blockers that were claimed to be of use in a variety of heart conditions. Again the miraculous effects were tempered by the development of such serious side-effects in one of them, Practolol, that the drug was withdrawn. At the same time, these drugs were found to have no effect upon the ultimate prognosis of the heart condition, in other words it was doubtful that they actually prolonged the life of the patient.

The next great 'wonder' drugs of the 1970's (and ultimately the 1980's), are the Prostaglandins, which are claimed to control just about every function in the body. They probably do, but their potency is so great and their effects upon the body so varied that warnings about them are already appearing in medical literature.

If we are willing to accept that these drugs are examples of therapeutic agents that have a wide variety of curative effects, why cannot vitamin E be accepted on the same principle? Medical literature abounds with reports of the effectiveness of the vitamin in many clinical conditions, yet these are largely ignored. Unlike most of the drugs in common use, vitamin E is both natural and safe. In fact, it is considered to be so lacking toxicity that, at the time of writing, the Department of Health and Social Security in the United Kingdom allow it to be sold without prescription and with no limit on potency!

WHY IS VITAMIN E SO CONTROVERSIAL?

The answer to this question must be partly in the fact that it is not possible to pin-point an exact medical condition associated with deficiency of the vitamin. With other vitamins, what happens in their deficiency is well established. For example, lack of vitamin B_1 causes beri-beri; that of nicotinamide produces pellagra and vitamin C deficiency gives rise to scurvy. Each of these diseases has well-defined clinical and biochemical symptoms that are reversed by treatment with the appropriate vitamin.

No specific disease has yet been associated with vitamin E deficiency so nutritionists and medical researchers happily assume that all of us are replete with the vitamin. Yet later we shall see how false this assumption is.

Another reason why vitamin E is not as widely used in medicine as it should be lies in its history. In the 1930's and 1940's the vitamin was being tested, and in many cases accepted, by various research centres throughout the world as a useful therapeutic agent. Then came the vast post-war research programme that produced drugs aimed at specific complaints. Therapy switched from prevention of disease to treatment, without worrying too much about what the cause was in the first place. The beneficial effects of vitamin E, both as a preventive as well as a curative treatment, tended to be overshadowed by these new developments.

Fortunately, despite these advances, the Shute Institute in Canada persevered with their treatment of heart conditions with vitamin E. Now, some thirty years later, more than 40,000 patients treated by them have benefited from vitamin E. Is it likely that such a high success rate is the result of chance?

MEGAVITAMIN THERAPY WITH VITAMIN E
The Shute treatment with vitamin E relies upon the concept that very large quantities of a vitamin act in a different way from the small amounts present in food. It is the therapeutic megavitamin approach to disease and it usually helps in specific degenerative diseases. All this means is that many illnesses are the result of a gradual degeneration, or dying, of a particular organ or part of the body, and this degeneration can often be traced to dietary causes.

If there is a mild deficiency of essential vitamins

like vitamin E over many years, the body will
gradually suffer and eventually a medical condition
will result. The only way to repair the ravages
induced by this long-term deficiency is to give
massive doses of the deficient vitamin in an attempt
to reverse the degenerative process. No diet can do
this on its own since the quantities present in food
are not sufficient to overcome prolonged mild
deficiency.

Obviously if enough vitamins were taken in the
diet throughout life, many such conditions would
not develop. We can now look at how dietary
changes over the years have contributed to a
deficiency of vitamin E in many of the population.
This deficiency in turn is related to the increase in
the degenerative diseases associated with modern
living.

DISEASES FROM DEFICIENCY

Coronary thrombosis was almost unknown before
1912. Further evidence that heart disease is of recent
origin is the observation by Sir Maurice Cassidy in
1946 that from 1926 to 1939, deaths from coronary
heart disease in Great Britain rose almost ten-fold
from 48 to 473 per million population. Sir Maurice,
who was Physician to King George VI, suggested
that 'The cause of coronary heart disease is still to
seek ... although an increasing number of
investigators relate it to nutritional deficiency of long
duration!'

Why has coronary thrombosis increased so
dramatically in the last 70 years or so? Likely factors
have included the softness of drinking water. There
has been a great increase in the intake of refined
carbohydrates, particularly white sugar. Chlorin-
ation of drinking water has been implicated.
So has the vast increase in the numbers of food

additives and the increasing pollution of our atmosphere with heavy metals. However, there is a growing belief that while these factors may be contributory to a minor degree, the basic reason lies in the deficiency of vitamin E over the years. Why particularly vitamin E?

It is because the development of a thrombosis or blood clot can be due to deficiency of a natural anti-clotting factor in the blood. Vitamin E is known to have the property of preventing the blood from clotting. If the chances of suffering from coronary thrombosis increased after 1912 it is not unreasonable to suppose that after this date changes in dietary habits induced a slow decline in blood vitamin E levels, since it is obtained only from the food we eat. The evidence that vitamin E intake from modern diets is declining is now overwhelming.

WHY WE LACK VITAMIN E

The most fundamental changes in our dietary habits since 1912 have been the refining of wheat, the removal of vitamins and minerals during food processing, the growing use of food additives and the pollution of the air, water and particularly the soil from which all food eventually arises.

As an example, let us look at what happens when white bread is produced. The wheat germ is removed from the grain before grinding and with it go 87 per cent of the gross minerals and 88 per cent of the trace minerals. The flour produced is then bleached to make it white and this process neatly disposes of the rest of the vitamin E.

Some vitamins B_1 and B_2 and nicotinamide are added to this emasculated flour, together with iron and calcium, but nothing else is replaced. As well as bread, other grains such as maize, wheat, oats and rice lose up to 90 per cent of their vitamin E when processed into breakfast foods.

The vitamin is removed from natural vegetable oils by physical refining, or destroyed by chemical hydrogenation or hardening to produce margarines, soft or otherwise. Deep freezing causes a lowering in vitamin E potency of foods. Today there are more than 3,000 additives allowed in food and many of these contribute to the destruction of vitamin E. An increased intake of polyunsaturated fatty acids without the concomitant increase in vitamin E can cause depletion of the body stores of the vitamin.

Little wonder then that all these changes in dietary habits since the early part of the century have contributed to a gradual decline in our intake of vitamin E. The parallel increase in the incidence of heart and blood circulation diseases is likely to be more than coincidental.

Dr A.L. Tappel, Professor of Food Science, Technology and Nutrition at the University of California at Davis is one of the foremost vitamin E researchers. He stated in an article on vitamin E in *Nutrition Today* (1973): 'While few compelling uses have been found for vitamin E, the more research is done on the substance, the more intriguing it appears. Thus, there is the nagging suspicion that there is a very important use for the vitamin and we are just not smart enough to see it!'

This statement may sum up the academics' attitude to vitamin E, but the following chapters will indicate the vast amount of knowledge that has been accumulated about the vitamin. More importantly, they will explain just how the vitamin has helped many people when used as a therapeutic agent, as well as a dietary supplement to ensure against deficiency. The evidence is here, there is no doubt about that. Perhaps by the end of the book you will find that vitamin E is not so controversial after all!

CHAPTER ONE

THE DISCOVERY AND PROPERTIES OF VITAMIN E

During experiments carried out in 1922 at the University of California, three research scientists, Evans, Scott and Bishop, fed rats an experimental diet of casein, cornstarch, lard, butter and yeast. The diet appeared to be adequate as the rats grew well and mated as often as rats fed on a control, normal diet. Nor was there any difficulty with the reproductive process. However it was noted that the rats showed a low fertility on the first generation and by the second they were wholly sterile. The pregnant females were found to have resorbed their foetuses which means that instead of carrying their litters to term, they were re-absorbing them back into their bodies. They were unable to give birth to their offspring.

Resorption of foetuses is a phenomenon quite common in the animal kingdom and it is generally thought to be a protective mechanism adopted by nature to prevent the birth of unhealthy offspring. In the higher animals like man, resorption is less common but the process of spontaneous abortion is believed to represent a similar protective mechanism. This phenomenon had been initiated in the experimental rats by the diet the animals were fed upon and it became obvious that the diet lacked some essential nutrient or nutrients. Further feeding experiments established that the addition of either lettuce, wheat germ or dried alfalfa leaves prevented the deficiency giving rise to resorption, allowing the rats to give birth to healthy offspring. Corroborative studies carried out elsewhere at the University of Arkansas by Dr B. Sure indicated that bean pods, polished rice, rolled oats, yellow maize and certain vegetables also supplied the nutrients necessary to prevent resorption.

THE 'FERTILITY VITAMIN'?

The only known vitamins in 1922 were vitamins A, B, C and D, so Dr Sure proposed calling the new essential nutrient vitamin E. Since it was associated with the property of allowing normal birth in rats it was dubbed the 'fertility vitamin', a name that has persisted to this day. When male rats were fed on the same deficient diet they became sterile and (as in the case of the females), the condition could be reversed by the same foods that allowed normal birth of baby rats.

Not surprisingly, these results caught the public's imagination and many men and women who suffered from low fertility or sterility saw hope in this new vitamin. Despite some successes, vitamin E has not turned out to be the long-sought panacea for these conditions in man although the association between vitamin E and sexual activity has remained. As we learn more about the mode of action and functions of vitamin E in the body, however, it is becoming apparent that the vitamin does have a connection with sexual function, albeit indirectly. It is likely that vitamin E is only one link in the chain of biochemical reactions that determines the efficiency of sexual function in the individual.

PROPERTIES

What was not realized at the time of the vitamin's demonstration in foods was that these foods only possessed a beneficial effect when used fresh. Conflicting results arose among various research groups because stale foods caused rancidity of the oils and fats leading to widespread destruction of the vitamin E. The confusion was not resolved until Evans and his associates isolated the pure vitamin from wheat germ oil in 1936. During the succeeding years the chemical structure of the vitamin was worked out and it was given the chemical generic name of tocopherol. This is derived from the Greek words *tokos* – birth and *phero* – to bear and means literally 'to bring forth offspring'. Once the chemical structure was known it merely became a matter of time before the compound was synthesized in the chemical laboratory. When this happened in 1939 it meant that meaningful amounts of the vitamin became available for the first time and research on it really got under way.

THE FAMILY OF TOCOPHEROLS

The term 'vitamin E' was used originally to denote the compound isolated from vegetable oils that was essential to maintain fertility in the rat. Subsequent investigation indicated that several naturally-occurring substances also possessed vitamin E activity and eventually it became obvious that at least four tocopherols occur in nature. These were isolated and identified and then designated alpha- beta- gamma- and delta-tocopherols. Despite only slight chemical differences the biological activity of all four is substantially different. If alpha-tocopherol is regarded as 100 per cent, the biological activities of the others are: beta-tocopherol 40 per cent; gamma-tocopherol 8 per cent and delta-tocopherol only 1 per cent when measured in the female rat resorption test. During the last fifteen years, a further four members of the tocopherols have been discovered. These are alpha- beta- gamma- and delta-tocotrienols. Although chemically related to the tocopherols, they show even less biological activity, the highest of which is alpha-tocotrienol with only 20 per cent of the potency of alpha-tocopherol. The term vitamin E is now reserved as a generic term for any tocopherol and tocotrienol derivatives having qualitatively the biological activity of alpha-tocopherol. In popular parlance, however, it continues to be synonymous with the most important member of the group alpha-tocopherol.

Although delta-tocopherol possesses only 1 per cent of the biological activity of alpha-tocopherol when measured in the rat resorption test it is claimed to be the most potent of all the tocopherols in its anti-oxidant function (i.e. prevention of rancidity in fats). Such differences reflect the wisdom of eating a diet containing all the tocopherols since it could be dangerous to assess the activity of a group of vitamins simply on one criterion, namely the rat resorption test.

HOW NATURAL AND SYNTHETIC VITAMIN E DIFFER

During the early period of research into vitamin E, the material was obtained from natural sources and many studies were carried out on this. When the synthetic material became available it was noted that on a gram for gram basis, this was less potent in terms of biological activity than the natural vitamin. The difference relates solely to chemical structure. Many substances exist in two forms which may be regarded for simplicity as right- and left-handed forms. The right-handed one is designated d- and the left-handed l-. When both types are possible, nature always chooses one and only one. There is no hard and fast rule about this, for example natural vitamin C is l-ascorbic acid; natural pantothenic acid is the d- form; natural amino acids are always of the l- type and natural vitamin E is always d-alpha-tocopherol, d-beta-tocopherol and so on.

If you regard your two hands with finger tips touching, each hand looks like the mirror image of the other. The only way they can be superimposed is palm to palm. It is impossible to cover one completely with the other in any other way. Hence although both hands have the same number of fingers, the same shape, the same size, they are essentially different in their relationship to one another. Similarly with certain substances. They look alike chemically with the same number of atoms and a similar structure but are different in the spatial relationships of these atoms. They are called isomers. Nature is very selective and can usually only use one of these isomers for its biological functions. The right hand will fit comfortably only into a right-handed glove. With difficulty it can be forced into a left-handed glove but its efficiency is impaired. Similarly a right-handed vitamin like d-alpha tocopherol will only fit into a right-handed body receptor where it can take part in its many functions. These receptors will reject a left-handed vitamin simply because it does not fit so that the wrong kind of vitamin isomer has no place in body metabolism usage.

Nature is not only selective in which isomer it can use but also in which isomer it can produce. Hence the natural one is always the active one. A chemist cannot be as selective. In synthesizing a vitamin that exists in two forms, the chemical reactions employed have an equal chance of going either way so that a mixture consisting of 50 per cent of each form results. This is known in the case of vitamin E as dl-alpha-tocopherol, which is called a racemic mixture. There are complicated methods of resolving these two forms in the laboratory to isolate the d-alpha one but economically it is not feasible. It is easier to let nature produce the correct type and then extract it from natural sources. Usually the body is unable to utilize the non-natural isomer, so it is rejected. It is not dangerous, merely useless. Out of a dose of 100mg of dl-alpha-tocopherol taken orally, the body will usefully employ the 50mg of d-alpha-tocopherol. The remaining 50mg of l-alpha-tocopherol cannot be used by the body and so is discarded and eventually excreted. The body is more efficient at resolving dl-alpha-tocopherol than is the chemist. When natural d-alpha-tocopherol is eaten, either as a supplement or in the diet, all of it is available to the system.

MILLIGRAMS AND INTERNATIONAL UNITS

Measurement of vitamins in International Units (I.U.) is a hangover from the early days of vitamin research. I.U.'s are a means of expressing the potency of vitamins in terms of biological activity. In the case of vitamin E, an I.U. is defined as the amount of vitamin E required to be given orally to vitamin E-deficient pregnant rats to prevent resorption of the foetus in 50 per cent of those rats. As the chemical structure of the E vitamins became known and as the vitamins were obtained in a pure state, it became possible to express them in terms of weight as milligrams. However, because of the differing biological potencies of the members of the vitamin E group, it is not possible to compare them with each other simply on a weight for weight basis. Biological activity must be taken into account. One milligram of d-alpha-tocopherol is more active in the animal system than one milligram of dl-alpha-tocopherol. Hence, one I.U. is now defined as equivalent to 1.00mg of dl-alpha-tocopheryl acetate or 1.10mg dl-alpha-tocopherol or 0.73mg d-alpha-tocopheryl acetate or 0.81mg d-alpha-tocopherol.

To put it another way:

1mg of dl-alpha-tocopheryl acetate	= 1 i.u.
1mg of dl-alpha-tocopheryl succinate	= 0.89 i.u.
1mg of d-alpha-tocopherol	= 1.1 i.u.
1mg of d-alpha-tocopheryl acetate	= 1.36 i.u.
1mg of d-alpha-tocopherol	= 1.49 i.u.
1mg of d-alpha-tocopheryl succinate	= 1.21 i.u.

The figures show that a milligram of natural d-alpha-tocopherol is almost 50 per cent more potent than a milligram of synthetic dl-alpha-tocopheryl acetate in terms of biological activity. Expressing vitamin E as I.U.'s is the only meaningful way of assessing the potency of a food or dietary supplement.

VITAMIN E ESTERS

In foods, vitamin E occurs as the free tocopherols yet in supplements, the vitamin is usually present as tocopheryl acetate or tocopheryl succinate. There is a very good reason for this. Pure tocopherols, when isolated from natural sources, are clear, odourless, quite viscous yellow oils. They are slowly destroyed by atmospheric oxygen and darken on exposure to light. This instability gives them only a limited shelf-life, even when encapsulated in a soft gelatine capsule. For these reasons the isolated free tocopherols are converted to esters with natural organic acids. D-alpha-tocopheryl acetate is a combination of d-alpha-tocopherol with acetic acid; d-alpha-tocopheryl succinate or d-alpha-tocopheryl acid succinate is the vitamin combined with succinic acid. Both these combinations (called esters) while retaining the biological activity of tocopherols, presents the vitamin in a much more stable form. The following table (Table 1) illustrates the greater stability of the tocopheryl acetate in vegetable oils when it was added before being subjected to high temperatures. The studies were carried out at the Company of Hoffman-la Roche of New Jersey, U.S.A., one of the world's largest producers of vitamin E.

Table 1 – The Effect of High Temperatures on Tocopherol and its Acetate

	Initial Tocopherol Content (mg per cent)	Per cent Tocopherol destroyed	Per cent Tocopheryl acetate destroyed
Unhydrogenated Corn Oil	100	97	13
Hydrogenated Corn Oil	105	99	19
Unhydrogenated Cotton Seed Oil	91	97	19
Hydrogenated Cotton Seed Oil	80	99	8
Unhydrogenated Soya Bean Oil	101	96	12
Hydrogenated Soya Bean Oil	73	99	13
Stabilized Safflower Oil	59	97	6
Unstabilized Safflower Oil	36	98	5

Although the temperatures used here were far in excess of ordinary cooking temperatures, the figures illustrate the stability of vitamin E acetate to light and heat.

When these esters of vitamin E, d-alpha-tocopheryl acetate and d-alpha-tocopheryl succinate are eaten the enzymes of the digestive system rapidly remove the acetate and succinate portions leaving the free tocopherols, which are absorbed as such. The acetate and succinate are then utilized in the energy-producing mechanisms of the body, so that nothing is wasted. When vitamin E is added to fortify vegetable oils or is presented in soft gelatine capsules it is usually d-alpha-tocopheryl acetate. In tablets it tends to be used as d-alpha-tocopheryl succinate, because this preparation is less oily and more suited to a dry tablet mix. However it is taken, only the presence of the d-alpha designation will ensure you are receiving the most biologically potent form of the vitamin.

ABSORBING VITAMIN E FROM FOOD

Vitamin E is a fat-soluble vitamin which means that it will dissolve in oils (both vegetable and mineral), fats, alcohol, chloroform and acetone. It is not soluble in water. Vitamin E is part of the unsaponifiable fraction of fats, in other words, when presented in the food it is not degraded to simpler units like oils and fats are by the digestive enzymes. When taken as a supplement in the form of the tocopheryl acetate or succinate, the acetic acid or succinic acid is removed by those enzymes but no further breakdown takes place. The important stage in digestion is reduction of the vitamin to very small oil particles.

This process of emulsification is achieved with the aid of bile salts which disperse the oily vitamin to such tiny droplets that direct absorption into the small intestine is possible. From here the vitamin eventually reaches the blood stream and so is distributed throughout the body. It is stored chiefly in the liver and in the fatty tissues of the body.

The vitamin reaches it maximum level in the body some 4 to 9 hours after being eaten. A balance is eventually reached between the level in the body and that taken in the diet and it is important to maintain body levels since the vitamin is steadily excreted via the bile and faeces. As much as several grams of vitamin E may be stored in the body, so a gross deficiency is unlikely in anyone on a good diet.

This does not however preclude an insidious subliminal mild deficiency developing when intake is lower than loss over a period of time. The two most important factors contributing to low vitamin E levels are (1) a low food intake due to a bad diet or destruction of the vitamin in the diet by over-cooking or over-processing and (2) the inability to absorb the vitamin efficiently. These factors will be dealt with in more detail later in the book.

WHY VITAMIN E CANNOT ALWAYS BE ABSORBED

Many people find that they cannot tolerate fats and oils for a variety of reasons including gall-bladder and liver dysfunctions, intestinal surgery or a deficiency of bile salts. Habitual taking of liquid paraffin as a laxative can trap the vitamin E (and indeed other fat soluble vitamins) in the mineral oil, making it unavailable for absorption.

Some people find that any oils or fats produce nausea so they tend to keep their intake down. For these reasons, vitamin E has now been produced in a water-solubilized (or capable of being dispersed by water) form that overcomes many of these problems. The process involves dispersing the vitamin E into the extremely small particles required for absorption by using a natural emulsifier. When this emulsified vitamin is added to water, a clear solution is produced, indicating complete solution of the oil.

This means that absorption can take place without the involvement of bile salts, since the vitamin is being presented to the intestine in the final stage of digestion. The water retains the vitamin so that liquid paraffin is unable to remove and dissolve it. Since this preparation by-passes the usual fat digestive system it is absorbed as a water-soluble vitamin, which often helps those suffering from malabsorption syndromes.

A water-solubilized preparation of vitamin E is now recommended by the medical profession for use in children as well as in premature babies who are particularly susceptible to vitamin E deficiency. A word of warning however; anyone suffering from fat malabsorption should be under medical supervision. Vitamin E is only one of the essential fatty compounds affected by this disease and the inability to digest and absorb fat can be indicative of many medical conditions.

HOW MUCH DO WE NEED?

No one knows with certainty how much vitamin E is required on a daily basis, simply because there is no single deficiency symptom that can be assessed. The usual criterion is the blood level of the vitamin but this is not a technique available to the layman. The statement is often made by official bodies that there is no deficiency because the vitamin is widely distributed in foods. Unfortunately this does not take into account destruction of the vitamin during food processing, including cooking, individual requirements or the varying proportions of the less biologically potent members of the group in the foods that are eaten. Nevertheless, attempts have been made to assess the daily needs of the vitamin in various groups of the population but these must be taken only as a guide.

The studies of Dr M.K. Horwitt in the United States reported in the American Journal of Clinical Nutrition in 1960 provide our best estimate of the vitamin E requirement of man. He established that a person's requirement is directly related to the body content of polyunsaturated fatty acids (PUFA) which in turn depends upon the dietary intake of these essential fatty acids.

The sources of PUFA are the vegetable oils such as sunflower, safflower and corn oils. An intake of corn oil supplying 16.5g linoleic acid which is the most important of these PUFA needed a simultaneous intake of 20 i.u. of d-alpha-tocopherol to just maintain blood tocopherol levels. Doubling the intake of linoleic acid to 33g required twice the quantity of vitamin E to maintain blood concentration of the vitamin at the same level. The average daily intake of PUFA in the United States is 24g so 30 i.u. of vitamin E activity would be expected to suffice daily.

Later studies by the same group in 1962 indicated that when 33g per day linoleic acid was included in the diet, stopping the vitamin E intake of 41 i.u. resulted in a rapid decrease of the vitamin concentration in the blood. The accumulation of vitamin E in the tissues had not kept pace with the accumulation of linoleic acid and the reserves of the vitamin were not available.

When other subjects were fed 4.5 i.u. of tocopherol per day for 54 months, an additional daily supplement of 20 i.u. was only partially effective in restoring blood levels of the vitamin. When a supplement of 82 i.u. was fed, this was completely effective in restoring normal blood concentrations of tocopherols.

The conclusion to be reached from such studies is

that an increase in PUFA intake should be paralleled by an increase in vitamin E intake of similar proportions. With present day publicity encouraging a higher intake of PUFA for many of the population, it is necessary to be aware of the importance of higher intakes of vitamin E. Theoretically, as vitamin E occurs in nature associated with vegetable oils that are the best sources of PUFA, both essential nutrients should increase together. However modern processing of oils does not always preserve the vitamin E and imbalance may occur.

A supplemental intake of 100 i.u. of vitamin E should be regarded as the absolute minimum for anyone who switches from saturated animal fats to unsaturated vegetable fats and oils. Even when the unsaturated fat diet is discontinued, supplementation with vitamin E should continue because the vitamin is lost from the body at a faster rate than are the PUFA. Stopping the supplemental vitamin E can easily induce a temporary deficiency in the body.

VITAMIN E REQUIREMENTS

Recommended allowances of vitamin E for the various sectors of the population can be summed up thus:

Low Birth Infants: The alpha-tocopherol content of human milk is between 2 and 5 i.u. per litre and may be considered adequate. Commercial formulas may not necessarily be satisfactory, particularly with the modern switch to higher unsaturated fatty acid levels. A level in milk of 4.5 i.u. of alpha-tocopherol per litre is a satisfactory intake when the milk contains 3.5 per cent of fat and *pro rata*.

Infants: The vitamin E intake of 3 to 5 i.u. per litre from human milk maintained a steady rise in blood vitamin-content so this quantity may be deemed to be sufficient up to the age of one year (9kg body weight).

Children: The requirements for vitamin E will increase with increasing body weight up to maturity, although the rate of growth slows down as this stage is reached. An intake increasing from 5 i.u. daily at 9kg body weight to 12 i.u. at 40kg body weight should be satisfactory in diets providing 4 to 7 per cent of calories as linoleic acid.

Adults: In order to maintain blood tocopherol levels, an intake of about 20 i.u. is needed and this should be provided by a calorie intake of 1800-3000 k. calories. During pregnancy and lactation the increased calorie intake should normally be accompanied by sufficient vitamin E to compensate for the amount deposited in the foetus and secreted in the milk.

The figures quoted above are taken from Official Recommended Daily Allowances suggested by the U.S. Government. The quantities must be regarded in their true light as average adequate intakes in balanced diets in the United States but tempered with the statement that 'there can be no single recommended value for each age and sex group'. No figures are quoted by the U.K. authorities. Realistic intakes of vitamin E will be discussed later in the book when dietary sources are considered.

CHAPTER TWO

DEFICIENCIES AND HOW TO OVERCOME THEM

The symptoms of vitamin E deficiency in rats are sterility in the males and the inability to give birth to offspring in pregnant females. The vitamin therefore has a fundamental role in the reproduction process in rats. Other species of animals were studied in a similar manner and it soon became obvious that many of their body functions were affected by lack of vitamin E but the manifestations varied depending upon the animal. The symptoms did not appear to have any common factor linking them with a possible function of the vitamin.

What is of interest is that in all experimental animals, the deficient condition always lasts a long time and the deficiency disease only very rarely leads to the death of the animal.

These findings may account for the fact that in man, little or no clinical vitamin E deficiency symptoms have been established with certainty. Deficiency states in farm animals are important since they frequently appear quite suddenly, presenting varied disease pictures. The effect of a deficient supply of vitamin E is made much worse if, in addition, there is a deficiency of protein or selenium or if large amounts of unsaturated fats, unsupplemented with the vitamin, are also administered.

It is important to study the symptoms of deficiency in animals since the conditions produced often resemble some diseases which humans are prone to suffer from. This does not mean that the known illness is necessarily due to vitamin E deficiency but often we find that such illnesses respond to vitamin E. The various complaints that animals suffer from in E deficiency will now be reviewed and their possible relationship to human disease will become apparent.

THE NERVOUS SYSTEM

The nervous system can be affected when vitamin E intake is restricted and it happens particularly in poultry which develop a disease called encephalomalacia. This is a softening of the brain substance due to thrombosis or some similar blockage with resulting lack of blood supply to the brain and subsequent degeneration. It is known as 'Crazy Chick Disease' and is characterized by the inability of the bird to hold its head upright. Mental confusion in the elderly person is often associated with low vitamin E levels, although other vitamin deficiencies may also contribute to it.

BODILY AND HEART MUSCLES

A muscle-wasting disease that resembles muscular dystrophy in man can be produced in the chick and in the rabbit by a tocopherol-deficient diet. It can be reversed by feeding vitamin E or delayed by reducing the quantities of polyunsaturated fatty acids in the E-deficient diet. Although skeletal muscle is affected by the vitamin deficiency in all domestic animals and livestock, the heart muscle is particularly weakened in pigs, calves and lambs, leading to sudden heart failure.

Low vitamin E is often a feature of people dying from heart attacks but no definite causal relationship has yet been found. Muscular dystrophy is not usually found in persons deficient in tocopherol nor is the disease of muscular dystrophy always improved by tocopherol therapy. However, Dr John Vester of the University of Pittsburgh reported that some sufferers from muscular dystrophy have been helped by massive doses of vitamin E but only in those cases where the fault could be traced to a lack of absorption of the vitamin.

BODY FAT

The development of 'yellow fat disease' is characteristic of vitamin E deficiency in mink, fox, cat, pig and poultry. The fatty tissues of the body contain fat that is yellow in colour instead of the usual 'pearly white'. Yellowing is due to increased oxidation (or rancidity) of body fat because the protective action of tocopherol has been lost.

A study from the Yale (USA) School of Medicine showed that a similar condition exists in vitamin E-deficient man where yellow fat is deposited in all smooth muscle. In the bowel this gives rise to the condition known as 'Brown bowel'. These findings are often observed at postmortem on patients who have died from heart disease, suggesting that the condition, at least in part, is associated with low vitamin E levels.

A similar yellow fat deposition occurs in every child with cystic fibrosis dying over the age of five but never in those less than two years of age. This suggests that the particular symptom of 'yellow fat disease' only appears after at least two years of vitamin E lack. Deficiency of vitamin E is often a feature of cystic fibrosis.

HOW DEFICIENCY AFFECTS THE BLOOD

Typical deficiency symptoms affecting the blood and circulatory systems in rats and pigs are a shortened life of red blood cells, which show a marked tendency to collapse, releasing their contents into the blood stream. When this happens over a long period, anaemia results. Anaemia is common in vitamin E-deficient apes and, of course, in man.

THE SKIN

A disease characterized by abnormal functioning of the skin and mucous membranes (i.e. mouth, eyes, vagina, anus), resulting in eczema, urticaria and itching occurs in poultry that are lacking vitamin E in the diet. At the same time there are frequent respiratory infections leading to catarrh of these mucous membranes and occasionally cancerous growth.

The disease is called exudative diathesis and it is also found in children. Although the condition is prevented and reversed by vitamin E supplementation in poultry, there appears to be no relationship between vitamin E deficiency and its occurrence in children. There is little doubt, however, that vitamin E can have a beneficial effect upon the skin and mucous membranes in man, so the relationship between the conditions in the two species may be closer than was originally thought.

REPRODUCTION

The effect of vitamin E deficiency upon the reproductive systems of both male and female rats has been mentioned but many other species are similarly affected. Degeneration of the testes occurs in piglets, calves, poultry and dogs when on an E-deficient diet. Female pigs, like rats, show a similar phenomenon, namely, the inability to give birth when lacking the vitamin.

New-born offspring of pigs, sheep and cows all show signs of debility and muscular degeneration when born with low vitamin E levels. Lack of vitality appears to be a constant feature of vitamin E deficiency in all species studied, including man.

DEFICIENCY SYMPTOMS

The studies mentioned above were carried out on animals in the hope of gaining a clue to similar diseases in man which may have been related to vitamin E deficiency but hopes are not completely realized. In adult man severe restriction of the dietary intake of vitamin E for lengths of time up to several years causes no clear-cut symptoms or signs. It is therefore possible for an insidious deficiency to develop with no obvious signs, apart from a generalized lack of vitality. Laboratory tests are available to indicate a deficiency but these can only be carried out using complicated and costly equipment.

One constant feature of deficiency is a low blood level of vitamin E. Another is an increased tendency for the red blood cells to burst. A third is excessive excretion of a compound called creatine in the urine. The level of creatine reflects the extent of muscle wasting – the more that is excreted, the more badly affected are the muscles. Children suffering from muscular dystrophy invariably have excess creatine in their urine.

THE BLOOD

Red blood cells must keep their shape to function correctly and anything that weakens the cell wall can lead to rupture of that cell. When this happens, the haemoglobin spills out of the cell and it can no longer function as an oxygen carrier. The red blood cells are then said to be haemolysed. The fragility of red blood cells is measured by noting how stable they are in the presence of weak hydrogen peroxide.

Hydrogen peroxide is not just a bleaching agent but is produced by the cells of the body during normal respiration. It is harmful when left undisturbed but there are mechanisms in the body cells for converting it to water and oxygen. Vitamin E is essential for this protective action so a lack of it allows the poisonous peroxide to build up.

Lack of vitamin E makes the red blood cells weak; supplementing with the vitamin strengthens them. Naturally a weakened red blood cell is more likely to be disrupted by the hazards it encounters while circulating throughout the body. As the number of weakened red blood cells that burst is increased, an anaemia develops that is associated purely with vitamin E deficiency.

The life of a normal red blood cell is 120 days but in vitamin E deficiency this is considerably shortened. A shorter life means that regeneration of new red blood cells must take place more rapidly and efficiently. Hence a strain is thrown upon the blood production mechanisms and when these cannot cope, anaemia results. This is known as haemolytic anaemia, which simply means that it is produced by an excessive breakdown of red blood cells.

VITAMIN E AND IRON IN ANAEMIA

If iron is taken when the anaemia is due to vitamin E deficiency, the condition gets worse. This is because, although ample or excess iron is available for blood formation, it cannot be incorporated into haemoglobin because vitamin E is lacking. As more red cells break down, more iron becomes available, the excessive concentration of the mineral inhibits further production of haemoglobin and a vicious circle is set up. Not every case of anaemia can be considered to be due to an iron deficiency and the possibility that it is due to lack of vitamin E should always be borne in mind. In the presence of sufficient vitamin E there is no harm in taking supplemental iron. It is only when the vitamin is low that iron may have a deleterious effect.

Only laboratory tests can decide whether an anaemia case is due to iron or vitamin E deficiency. The safest course for the individual is an ample intake of vitamin E per day, as a supplement if necessary. This ensures that any anaemia that develops cannot be due to deficiency of the vitamin.

DEFICIENCIES IN BABIES AND CHILDREN

Premature babies are particularly susceptible to a haemolytic anaemia induced by vitamin E deficiency. Variable intakes by the mother during pregnancy and inefficient transfer of the vitamin across the placenta places the new-born baby in a precarious position. Many prematurely born babies are treated with high pressure oxygen during the first days of life and in the absence of vitamin E, such treatment may increase the risk of retrolental fibroplasia – a blinding disease involving obstruction of the retina or internal surface of the eye. This does not develop when the baby has normal levels of vitamin E.

Feeding the child with cows' milk may not help the deficient condition because, although the polyunsaturated fatty acid content is low, the d-alpha tocopherol content varies with the season, being particularly low in winter and early spring. A high level of unsaturated fat in artificial milks that are not supplemented with vitamin E can also cause a severe deficiency.

Human colostrum and early milk are very rich in tocopherol, so that breast-fed babies receive large amounts of vitamin E during the first few days of life. Most dried milks are now supplemented with vitamin E to compensate for variable levels and also because such milks usually have added iron. Vitamin E supplementation of artificially fed premature babies from the tenth day has been recommended. In Africa and the Far East, such treatment has been successful in preventing retrolental fibroplasia.

As the child is weaned off milk, this source of supplemental vitamin E is lost and the intake of the vitamin starts dropping again. A form of anaemia that responds only to vitamin E then develops, giving rise to a condition that is prevalent in children in the Middle and Far Eastern parts of the world. When this happens, the deficiency is often made worse by an excessive intake of iron from the cooking pots of those regions. The only treatment is increased intake of vitamin E, either from foods or supplements.

HOW DEFICIENCY DEVELOPS IN MAN

(i) *Inefficient absorption of fats:*

Persistent inability to absorb fats in the most likely mechanism by which adults become deficient in the fat-soluble vitamin E. The following conditions have all been found to reduce absorption, leading eventually to gross biochemical signs of deficiency.

Intestinal disease.

Pancreatic disease.

Following gastric or intestinal surgery.

Alcoholism.

Cirrhosis of the liver – due to reduced output of bile salts that are needed for absorbing the vitamin E.

Obstructive jaundice – due to the inability of the bile salts to enter the digestive tract.

Cystic fibrosis.

Tropical Sprue.

Coeliac disease.

The characteristic feature of all these conditions is steatorrhoea or the presence of excess fat in the faeces. The underlying complaint is the inability to absorb all fats, among which are the fat-soluble vitamins, including E.

Hence the varied signs and symptoms associated with steatorrhoea such as diarrhoea, weakness, ease of fatigue, lassitude, weight loss, poor appetite, pallor, bleeding tendencies, muscle cramps, bone pain and scaling of the skin are more the result of a generalized fat deficiency, although the lack of vitamins A, D, E and K must contribute to some of these.

In all cases studied there was a relationship between vitamin E deficiency and the individual's long term inability to absorb fats. The longer the condition persisted, the worse the deficiency became.

In all the above conditions, high potency supplements of vitamin E were able to restore the blood levels to normal. Superior results were obtained, however, when a water-solubilized form of the vitamin was taken, as this bypassed the usual fat absorption mechanisms.

(ii) *Excessive intake of polyunsaturated oils:*

In recent years the public have been aware of the benefits of replacing saturated animal fats with polyunsaturated oils (such as sunflower, safflower and maize oils) that are rich in the essential polyunsaturated fatty acids. A lowering of blood levels of cholesterol with subsequent decreased chances of developing heart disease have been amongst the benefits claimed. Yet this dietary change has long been known to be the best device for accelerating vitamin E deficiency in animals.

An 8-year long study carried out at the L.B.

Mandel Research Laboratory at the Elgin State Hospital, Illinois by Dr M.K. Horwitt and colleagues confirmed a similar effect in 38 weeks on male volunteers. They all developed vitamin E deficiency when fed vegetable oils without supplemental vitamin E. Vegetable oils vary in quality depending upon their vitamin E content, which may be high or low, depending upon the extraction procedures used. When such oils contain insufficient vitamin E to counterbalance the high concentration of polyunsaturated fatty acids, the deficit must be supplied either by other dietary components or by body reserves of the vitamin.

Hence the possibility cannot be ignored that an appreciable increase in consumption of such oils, whether as supplemental or replacement fats, could result in gradual depletion and eventual deficiency of vitamin E. The reason is that in protecting the polyunsaturated fatty acids from oxidation, the tocopherol itself is destroyed. Hence there is a sensitive balance between the polyunsaturated fatty acids requiring protection and the amount of tocopherol available to protect them.

The simple rule is to take extra vitamin E whenever the intake of vegetable oils is increased. Once these oils are absorbed into the body it is essential to ensure there is sufficient vitamin E to protect them inside the tissues. This is best done with supplemental vitamin E. One unit of natural vitamin E should be taken for every 2 grams of unsaturated oils or fats eaten.

(ii) *Excessive oxygen:*
Spacecrafts have carried an atmosphere of pure oxygen since these conditions were shown to help astronauts to withstand the fantastic acceleration required to break free of the earth's gravitational

pull. It has been known since 1935 that pure oxygen can be dangerous and this was confirmed when volunteers in simulated space capsules containing 100 per cent oxygen tended to develop convulsions and haemolytic anaemia. This was due to rancidity of the body polyunsaturated fatty acids in a condition usually prevented by vitamin E.

Just as an excessive supply of polyunsaturated fatty acids require additional vitamin E to protect them, so an abnormally large supply of oxygen would be expected to set up the same requirement. This hypothesis was first proved in mice, then confirmed in the space capsule volunteers, yet it was ignored in early space flights.

When Borman and Lovell made the Gemini 7 flight in December 1965 they were given normal freeze-dried diets which were later found to be barely adequate in vitamin E levels required for living under normal conditions. These crews lost between 20 and 30 per cent of their red blood cell mass during flight, leading to extensive haemolytic anaemia and fatigue. At the same time they suffered from a general weakening of the heart and blood circulation system.

When the Apollo II crew of Armstrong, Aldrin and Collins made their historic landing on the moon they had their freeze-dried foods supplemented with vitamin E and they suffered no red blood cell loss nor fatigue. The mental stress encountered on such hazardous flights was also reduced when extra vitamin E was added to the diet.

Most of us are never likely to encounter conditions of oxygen excess in normal lives but the experiences with space travellers emphasize the sensitivity of the body's reactions to mild tocopherol lack. How many modern diets can guarantee a constant, adequate supply of vitamin E?

(iv) *Mineral oils:*

Mineral oils such as liquid paraffin are widely used in relieving and preventing constipation. They work by simple lubrication and because they are not digested or absorbed as food oils are, they represent a seemingly innocuous treatment for constipation. However, liquid paraffin is able to dissolve vitamin E along with other fat soluble vitamins and because the oil is not digested or absorbed, the vitamins stay trapped in it, to be eventually excreted. Once vitamin E is dissolved in liquid paraffin there is no way the body can assimilate it.

The occasional use of such laxatives like liquid paraffin usually pose no problem as far as vitamin E is concerned. Unfortunately this oil is often the laxative of choice in chronic constipation where it may be taken daily for many months or even years. In such cases, the chances of developing vitamin E deficiency are increased. The only measures are (i) Take a vitamin E supplement at a meal when liquid paraffin is not taken. (ii) Take a natural laxative that does not include liquid paraffin (e.g. bran). (iii) Take the vitamin E supplement in a water-solubilized form that does not dissolve in the mineral oil. Remember that any laxative taken over a long period of time is not good practice. The cause of constipation should be looked for, rather than the treatment.

SIGNS AND SYMPTOMS OF DEFICIENCY

In the premature infant a syndrome (collection of symptoms) of irritability, oedema (retention of water in the tissues) and haemolytic anaemia may occur in association with low vitamin E body levels. Similar symptoms are presented in children and in all cases these signs and symptoms disappear with tocopherol supplementation. However, in adults, discrete signs of vitamin E deficiency are not readily observable by the individual. Often there is a simple lack of vitality which manifests itself in different ways. It may give rise to lethargy, apathy, inability to concentrate, irritability, disinterest in physical activity and decreased sexual performance. Muscle weakness can also be associated with low body levels of the vitamin.

No doubt the fact that vitamin E often helps in these situations suggests that the first line of treatment is supplementation with the vitamin. Most people suffer from one or more of these symptoms at some time in their lives and in a high proportion of cases, simple addition of vitamin E to their diets suffices to overcome the condition. When there is no response to the vitamin it is obvious that something else is at fault and other remedial steps can be taken.

The true measures of deficiency are biochemical parameters which can only be determined by laboratory tests. These are: (1) low blood levels of the vitamin; (2) increased fragility of red blood cells; (3) increased creatine in the urine (this indicates, and is a measure of muscle wasting); (4) haemolytic anaemia; (5) deposition of brown or yellow fat.

Those suffering from heart disease often show degeneration of the heart muscles with massive scarring and accumulations of brown pigment in their fat, suggesting a localized – if not general – vitamin E deficiency. Ceroid (brown or yellow pigment) deposition in tissues is permanent and although it is accepted as a sign of vitamin E deficiency, it is not known to cause any functional defect.

OFFICIAL REQUIREMENTS

It is difficult to assess the daily requirement of

vitamin E because the intake is dependent upon other dietary ingredients. These include polyunsaturated fatty acids (as in vegetable oils) sulphur-containing amino acids like cystine, cysteine and methionine and vitamin A. Vitamin E is required to protect both polyunsaturated acids and vitamin A so that, as the intake of these increases, so should that of vitamin E.

Similarly, there is an association of vitamin E with the quality of protein in the diet. Protein is simply a collection of units called amino acids, which are essential building-blocks of the body. A high quality protein is one containing a high proportion of the sulphur-containing amino acids and it requires more vitamin E than does a low quality protein. This is because the vitamin also has a protective influence on these compounds. Selenium is able to mimic vitamin E in some of its body reactions so as selenium intake rises, less vitamin E is required.

According to authoritative sources in the UK (*Recommended Intakes of Nutrients for the United Kingdom*, HMSO 1969), most diets supply 10 i.u. or more of vitamin E per day. Later estimates from USA sources (*Recommended Dietary Allowances, National Academy of Sciences*, 1974) suggest a daily intake of 10 to 20 i.u. per day in diets supplying between 1800 and 2000 calories. Whether such levels are sufficient is open to doubt but intakes from a good, all-round, balanced diet, believed to be up to 30 i.u. per day may be regarded as the absolute maximum from food.

Researchers used animal experiments to determine how little vitamin E is required to prevent the symptoms of deficiency, then extended the figures on a weight for weight basis to man. As we have seen however, deficiency symptoms in animals do not appear to relate to man so it is difficult to see the rationality of this approach. These figures together with those of typical diets have been combined in order to calculate a suggested daily allowance. This varies amongst different countries showing there is a true lack of knowledge concerning vitamin E intake. Nevertheless the figures suggested range from 5 i.u. for infants through 10 to 15 i.u. for children to a top intake of 30 i.u. for adults.

Such figures do not take into account several important factors: (1) variation of requirements among individuals; (2) losses during food processing such as cooking; (3) bio-availability which is simply a measure of how much of the vitamin that is eaten is actually absorbed and used by the body. Not allowing for these factors probably accounts for most of the conditions arising from vitamin E deficiency. Here we are referring, not to a gross deficiency which can give rise to the signs and symptoms referred to above, but to a mild deficiency that can eventually cause a gross deficiency when experienced over a number of years.

HOW TO TAKE SUPPLEMENTS
Vitamin E supplements, whether as tablets or capsules, should be taken with – or just after – meals. This will ensure maximum absorption and utilization of the vitamin. If taken on an empty stomach, the oily nature of the vitamin may cause nausea.

Simple supplementation to ensure against even a mild deficiency, without reference to dietary intake, should be a minimum of 100 i.u. Anyone who wishes to lessen the chances of heart attack or blood circulation problems can safely take up to 500 i.u. per day. Individuals who are aware of or have suffered from any of the conditions that vitamin E has helped, can take up to 1000 i.u. per day.

Anything above this should be under medical supervision, since the chances are that they are already suffering from a complaint that needs massive doses of the vitamin but these can vary depending upon their existing medical treatment. When on high doses of vitamin E, a person's condition should be regularly monitored by his practitioner.

Vitamin E has such a reaction upon many of the body processes that it is wise to start with a low level supplement and gradually build up to the high potency intake. This is so that its action is tempered and to avoid wasting the vitamin by over-excretion if this gradual build-up is ignored. A typical regime would be 100 i.u. per day for a month increasing to 250 i.u. for a further month and by similar steps up to 400 or 500 i.u. as a daily supplement.

One may stop and persevere at any level, whether it is for a transient condition like the menopause or a chronic complaint like diabetes or heart and blood circulation problems. Most vitamin E is taken as an insurance policy because people are now becoming aware of the possibility of an insidious deficiency developing as a result of the modern treatments of foods that can destroy the vitamin.

MEGAVITAMIN THERAPY

The second level of vitamin E supplementation is the therapeutic level, sometimes known as megavitamin therapy. This is medicinal treatment using vitamin E as a drug, since the quantities given are far above those obtainable from the diet. These doses range from 75 to 100 i.u. per day to treat premature babies suffering from oedema and haemolytic anaemia, up to 3500 i.u. or more given to patients suffering from heart and blood circulation disease.

There are two medical conditions where vitamin E

should not be taken in high doses. One is in rheumatic heart disease, where dosage is so critical that it requires medical supervision. The second is uncontrolled high blood-pressure. Where the blood pressure is already under the control of drugs, vitamin E is often helpful but the additive effects of the vitamin often means that the level of these drugs may be decreased. The only person to decide this is the medical or other practitioner. In fact, whenever any individual has been on self-medicated vitamin E in high dose, this should be mentioned to the practitioner.

After treating more than 35,000 patients with vitamin E over many years, Dr Evan Shute of the Shute Institute of Clinical and Laboratory Medicine in London, Ontario, has found no toxic effects with high doses of the vitamin, apart from the two exceptions mentioned above.

LARGER DOSES

When d-alpha tocopherol is administered orally in massive doses, it is well tolerated. No symptoms of toxicity have been reported in a number of species, including rats, mice, rabbits, dogs, cats and monkeys. An American study has been published by the American Chemical Society in 1957. Adult volunteers were given levels as high as 500 to 600 i.u. vitamin E per kg body weight on a daily basis for 5 months with no recognizable symptoms of toxicity. This represents a daily intake of about 40,000 i.u. for an average 70kg (11 stone) adult.

There are, however, uncontrolled observations of possible untoward effects of large doses of vitamin E in small numbers of human subjects. In man the reported effects have always been minor and have never led to severe and permanent defects. If any side effects do occur, these can always be associated with the high vitamin E intake and cessation or reduction of the dose invariably removes the symptoms. For example one report in the *New England Journal of Medicine* (1973) mentions that a dose of 800 i.u. per day for one week induced a weakness and fatigue in one person, rather like the symptoms of influenza. Reducing the intake to 400 i.u. per day caused no ill-effect and this dose was easily tolerated for long periods.

Other reports in the *Journal of the American Medical Association* (1974) found no ill-effects in a number of patients treated with 800 i.u. of the vitamin per day. At much larger doses there was reversible muscle weakness, disturbed reproductive functions and gastro-intestinal upsets.

Typical symptoms of vitamin E excess are muscle weakness and proneness to fatigue. Other signs of over-dosage include rising blood-pressure and palpitations of the heart. Sometimes the high concentration of oil gives rise to mild diarrhoea and nausea but these are not noted with the water-solubilized forms. Biochemical changes may cause the raised creatine level in the urine mentioned before.

Like other fat-soluble vitamins, the symptoms of vitamin E excess are similar to those of its deficiency. However, these are simply warning signs and a reduction of dosage to a level where these symptoms are not produced indicates that amount of vitamin E which the body can tolerate.

An Expert panel on Food Safety and Nutrition said in the publication *Food Technology* in 1977 'There is no evidence that the tocopherols are toxic, even in large doses'. A leading article in *The Lancet* in 1974 concluded that 'Vitamin E is a natural nutrient; administration leads to no toxic effects'.

In rare cases there may be an effect of vitamin E

upon other medical treatments. There is one case on record of a man having anticoagulant therapy for blood clotting problems, whose vitamin K levels decreased during therapy with 1200 i.u. of vitamin E per day. A low vitamin K concentration in the blood leads to an increase in the length of time it takes the blood to clot. Once the vitamin E was stopped, the concentration of vitamin K dependent coagulating factors returned to normal and a normal blood-clotting time was resumed. This effect indicates the anti-thrombotic (i.e. anti-blood clotting) property of vitamin E. Large doses of alpha tocopherol in anaemic children may suppress the normal blood-forming response to injected iron. This, however, represents no problem once the deficient factor causing the anaemia has been identified.

CHAPTER THREE

WHAT VITAMIN E DOES IN THE BODY

(i) *It reduces the oxygen requirements of muscles and organs*
All muscles and organs in the human body require oxygen to function efficiently. This is because oxygen is essential in the conversion of glucose to energy. The only way that oxygen can be supplied to the working parts of the body is via the blood where it is carried in the red blood cells attached to the red pigment called haemoglobin.

When a muscle is at rest, its oxygen requirements are minimal. As it is called upon to contract to produce movement, more energy is required and so more oxygen has to be supplied. This is achieved by an increase in the blood flow to that muscle. Vitamin E has the ability to decrease the needs of muscles and other tissues for that increased oxygen. In other words, in the presence of adequate vitamin E the muscle can carry out the same amount of work using less oxygen.

The vitamin performs this function in two ways. Firstly, it increases the efficiency of oxygen usage by the muscle. Secondly, it helps to protect the muscle against the harmful substances produced when glucose is converted into energy. The importance of the power of vitamin E becomes apparent when we consider what happens when the blood supply to a muscle such as the heart is curtailed.

Arteries are the blood vessels that supply blood, and hence oxygen, to all parts of the body. They can become narrowed for a variety of reasons, including thrombosis (a blood clot), atherosclerosis (thickening of the arterial wall due to deposition of fat) and arteriosclerosis (hardening and constriction of the arteries). Whatever the cause, this narrowing of the blood vessel decreases the blood supply to the heart or other organs. The veins carry oxygen towards the heart and when these become blocked, insufficient blood reaches the heart and stagnation results. In either case the muscles and organs suffer because they are receiving insufficient oxygen.

Once cells are deprived of oxygen they die. The role of vitamin E therefore is to enable these cells to function efficiently on less oxygen. It conserves the small amount of oxygen that is available and so helps preserve the life and usefulness of those cells. The famous Canadian doctors, the Shute brothers, who pioneered the treatment of heart disease with vitamin E, have taken photographs of organs that are suffering from a decreased blood supply. After treatment with vitamin E, further photographs have clearly indicated a regeneration of the dead area as a result of the conservation of available oxygen produced by the vitamin.

The heart muscle itself is supplied with blood by the coronary arteries. When these become blocked a heart attack is often the result, because of insufficient oxygen supply to that organ. A similar situation can arise in the brain where a blockage produces a stroke, since the brain is very sensitive to lack of oxygen. In the legs, similar constrictions cause the complaint known as intermittent claudication, where pain is produced on exercise because of lack of oxygen to the leg muscles.

In all these conditions, the Shute brothers and others have demonstrated the effectiveness of vitamin E in overcoming the effects of partial blockage of blood vessels.

(ii) *Vitamin E acts as an anti-blood clotting agent*

As long ago as 1946, the Shute brothers at their practice in Canada noted that vitamin E both dissolved fresh pre-formed blood clots and prevented their formation. It exerts its action by inhibiting the protein thrombin, which functions normally as a blood clot producer. The process of blood clotting is an essential defence mechanism against excessive bleeding that occurs when a blood vessel is cut. Thrombin is the normal blood constituent that controls this mechanism. It can however get out of hand and produce blood clots within blood vessels where they are not needed and the result is a thrombosis.

Many studies reported in the *Journal of the American Medical Association* in 1950, and further studies by Doctor Alton Ochsner and his group published in the *New England Journal of Medicine* in 1964 stressed the importance of vitamin E in dissolving and preventing blood clots. He states that 'alpha tocopherol is a potent inhibitor of thrombin that does not produce excessive bleeding and is therefore a safe preventative agent against thrombosis'.

Thrombin is not usually present as such in blood but it is normally formed from inactive precursors in the blood only when the blood-clotting mechanism is needed. In some diseases, however, thrombin is produced without any apparent reason and this is where the danger of thrombosis is increased. Vitamin E is always present in the blood and is thus available to act as an anti-thrombin when so required. If there is insufficient vitamin present, the dangers of blood-clot formation are increased. Adequate vitamin E is the best prevention against unwanted blood clots, which in turn cause such serious complaints as phlebitis, heart attacks and strokes. Dr Ochsner in the journal *Postgraduate*

Medicine in 1968 suggests that the increase in frequency of these fatal diseases is related to the relatively low intakes of the vitamin in modern times.

(iii) *Vitamin E opens up new channels of blood supply*

When a blood vessel becomes blocked either totally or partially, the body responds by opening up new blood vessels that bypass the constricted one and thus allow blood to flow to a muscle or organ again. The new system of blood vessels is known as the 'collateral circulation' and vitamin E speeds up its development. This function of the vitamin is very important indeed, because a constricted blood supply to any part of the body can result in the 'death' of that particular area.

Part of the use of vitamin E in treating heart attacks induced by thrombosis is due to this action. By stimulating the formation of alternative routes for blood to reach the heart, it allows this organ to carry on functioning. The effect is seen in heart patients by an improvement in clinical signs and increased tolerance for exercise. The efficiency of the heart's functioning is indicated by an electro-cardiogram (ECG) and this too is seen to improve in those patients who have suffered a heart attack and received subsequent treatment with vitamin E. The vitamin is a unique treatment in this respect, since it alone has the power to continually stimulate new blood supplies to affected organs.

(iv) *Vitamin E causes the smaller blood vessels to dilate (widen)*

Arteries and veins are the main blood vessels carrying blood to and from all parts of the body. They are wide and strong, since they work under great pressure. Eventually, however, they can narrow to arterioles (small arteries) and capillaries

which are the small vessels that actually bring blood
into contact with the tissues. Capillaries are the
junction between arteries bringing oxygen and
nourishment to the tissues and the veins that carry
away the waste products. The state of the capillaries
is thus particularly significant in determining how
much blood is going to eventually reach the organs
and tissues of the body. As they widen, more blood
becomes available. This is of great importance in the
healing of wounds and the regeneration of skin that
has been burned.

Vitamin E dilates the capillaries and ensures that
sufficient blood is available to help heal the damaged
area. Sometimes people who take a high dose of the
vitamin experience a transient flushing which is due
to dilation of the capillaries. It is harmless and
usually induces a feeling of well-being.

(v) *Vitamin E strengthens capillary walls*

Normally capillary walls are strong enough to contain the blood flowing in them but there are diseases
where these walls weaken and allow blood to seep
through. A simple bruise is the result of capillaries
being damaged by a blow and allowing blood to flow
into the surrounding area. Usually though,
abnormal capillary permeability is due to an
infection or an allergy. Infections, particularly in the
throat, sometimes lead to kidney disease where the
capillaries become permeable to blood constituents,
such as protein, that are usually retained.

Acute rheumatic fever is another complaint where
capillaries are damaged due to an infection and
allergic reaction. Dr Wilfred E. Shute has reported
many cases of acute kidney disease and acute
rheumatic fever which have responded very quickly
to treatment with vitamin E, allowing complete
recovery in 2 or 3 days. He has demonstrated that the

vitamin restores normal capillary permeability, allowing the damaged tissues to return to their healthy state. When the diseases are of long duration, however, alpha tocopherol is a less effective treatment.

(vi) *Vitamin E helps in regenerating new skin*

When the skin is broken for any reason, the body's defences are mobilized to repair the wound, since the skin is the main line of defence against infection. Vitamin E contributes a major role in repairing surface wounds and ulcers, probably by its action in stimulating an increased blood supply to the affected area. Many ulcers that have failed to heal under ordinary treatment have responded dramatically to a high oral dose of vitamin E. The ability of alpha tocopherol to limit cell death to those cells that have been killed by the burning agent has made the vitamin of particular value in treating burns.

Vitamin E inhibits the over-production of scar tissue and prevents scar contraction as wounds heal, a most important function. When they contract, large scars sometimes produce deformities which may necessitate skin grafts. Deformities can often be prevented by using vitamin E and the need for skin grafting can be overcome. Similarly, even old, long established scars and stretch marks can be removed with vitamin E treatment. Surgeons working on these problems at the Shute Institute have this advice, however. Treatment of wounds and removal of scars are more effective if vitamin E is applied in an ointment to the affected area as well as taken by mouth in tablet or capsule form.

(vii) *Vitamin E helps in the process of normal clotting of blood*

Many factors are concerned with the normal clotting

of blood that is an essential defence mechanism when blood vessels are cut. The ultimate process, however, is the production of a plug or blood clot that seals off the wound. The clot is made up of white blood cells called platelets. The mobilization of these cells when they are needed is under the control of vitamin E.

Abnormally low platelet levels in the blood leads to a condition called 'purpura' characterized by the purple patches under the skin. Vitamin E stimulates the production of these cells and normalizes their behaviour, so finding a role in the treatment of purpura.

Hence, vitamin E finds a role in both producing blood clots and in the dissolving of them (see (ii) above). However, this apparent paradox is explained by the different mechanisms operating for normal and abnormal blood clot formation. Normal blood clots are produced by the stimulus of the wound and vitamin E helps mobilize the platelets to form them.

Production of a blood clot or thrombosis inside the body is an abnormal condition and it is stimulated by other factors not connected with the normal blood clotting mechanism. Vitamin E then becomes the agent which dissolves these thromboses, or more importantly; helps to prevent them in the first place.

(viii) *Vitamin E improves the action of insulin in diabetes*
There are 46 papers in the medical literature confirming the value of alpha tocopherol in the treatment of diabetes. Dr V. Butturini of Milan has reported in Italian medical journals that some diabetics require less insulin after taking vitamin E. As many as 25 per cent of 'adequately' treated patients suffering from diabetes have decreased

insulin requirements, according to the Shute brothers.

What is important is that diabetes has two phases. The first is characterized by high blood sugar and is controlled by insulin injections or the oral drugs now in common use. The second is the involvement of the blood system that comes later, resulting in blindness, arteriosclerosis, high blood-pressure and gangrene. When vitamin E is taken at the first signs of diabetes, it functions in both phases. As well as reducing the requirement for insulin, it helps in preventing the onset of the blood circulation complications. According to Dr Evan V. Shute, 'Alpha tocopherol plugged the leak in the insulin boat!'

(ix) Vitamin E acts as a diuretic

Heart, kidney and liver diseases are often characterized by retention of water in the body, one of the obvious signs of which is swollen ankles (oedema). The main route for water disposal is through the kidneys, whence it is excreted as urine. Vitamin E stimulates the flow of urine by acting through the normal mechanisms of the kidneys. Although it is less powerful than many of the potent synthetic diuretic drugs available, it has the advantage of functioning in a natural manner. What is even more significant is that it exerts its action without the serious loss of minerals that is a side effect of the diuretic drugs.

(x) Vitamin E increases the power and activity of muscles

Many athletes can testify to the greater endurance, better stamina and improved well-being they experienced after vitamin E supplementation. Trials carried out by Mr Lloyd Percival of Canada's Sports

College demonstrated the effectiveness of vitamin E for improving athletic performance. He noted a lower increase of the pulse rate on exertion, with a quicker reversion to normal on resting. Less muscle fatigue and a faster recovery of ability to re-run a race were also associated with the taking of vitamin E according to Dr Lambert, the famous Irish veterinary surgeon.

In India, controlled trials indicated that alpha tocopherol seemed to increase the ability of soldiers at high altitude to march and carry heavier burdens without fatigue.

(xi) *Vitamin E acts as the 'Great Protector' of the body*
One of the most important functions of vitamin E is to protect other essential nutrients like vitamin A, vitamin C, vitamin F (the polyunsaturated fatty acids) and the sulphur-containing amino acids. This protective influence takes place not only in the food we eat but extends to these compounds when they are functioning in the body itself. Vitamin E protects because it is an anti-oxidant, that is, it prevents destruction of these essential components by oxygen.

A similar role is believed to explain the anti-ageing effect of vitamin E that has been demonstrated in animals by the studies of Dr A.L. Tappel at the Geriatric Studies Institute in the United States. The process of ageing is accelerated by the formation of 'free radicals'. These are highly reactive compounds that arise most frequently from the polyunsaturated fats that have been oxidized in various biochemical body reactions and usually disposed of by body defence mechanisms. When these 'free radicals' are allowed to build up to a high concentration, they can be very damaging to health. Vitamin E is believed to neutralize these 'free radicals' as part of its protective

function so it is important that adequate tocopherol
is always available.

Research at the University of California at Davis
has confirmed reports by others that vitamin E can
protect animals against the ill-effects of atmospheric
pollutants such as ozone, nitrogen dioxide, car
exhaust fumes and smog. Many of the basic features
of these animal tests are similar to conditions
affecting some human beings. It is highly likely that
the positive effects of vitamin E as a protective agent
against pollution apply also to man.

Vitamin E is also able to protect against the
harmful side-effects associated with the long-term
treatment with analgesics. Even simple pain killers
like aspirin, codeine and paracetamol can damage
the liver and kidneys when taken over long periods.
In animal experiments, vitamin E given in high doses
was proved to prevent the ill-effects of these drugs.

Recent reports in the *British Medical Journal* have
confirmed a similar role for vitamin E in man. High
oral intake of alpha tocopherol was able to neutralize
the harmful effects of large doses of paracetamol
when these were taken in attempts at self-poisoning.
This life-saving aspect of tocopherol is an exciting
development that may be extended to other poisons.

VITAMIN E AND SELENIUM: THE TWIN NUTRIENTS

Brief mention was made in section (ix) above of the
'Great Protector' role that has been assigned to
vitamin E. As a result of recent research it has now
become apparent that the trace mineral selenium
plays as important a role as the vitamin itself.
Moreover, both the two nutrients act as synergists.
This simply means that both working together have
a greater effect than the sum of their individual

effects. They potentiate the activity of each other, making each other more powerful.

In some of its functions selenium can 'spare' vitamin E – for example a high concentration of the vitamin can exert a protective action on the heart but similar benefits are obtained with a lower potency of E if selenium is also supplemented. However, full realization of the protective roles of both compounds is best obtained when both are available at the same time and in adequate quantities. Then they function together almost as if they were a single nutrient.

The human body contains roughly 100 trillion cells. Each cell is continually under attack by highly reactive chemical compounds, the aforementioned 'free radicals'. These result directly or indirectly from radiation, atmospheric pollutants such as ozone, car exhaust fumes, tobacco smoke and smog and from some constituents of the diet. They are produced during normal metabolic body processes, particularly those involving oxidation. Oxidation means reaction with oxygen and it is vital for energy production under normal conditions. When it becomes uncontrolled under the influence of the 'free radicals' however, body processes start to go wrong. Normally the healthy body can cope with the 'free radicals' with the aid of vitamin E which captures them, thus sparing the cell structure which would otherwise be damaged. During the process vitamin E itself is destroyed which is why a constant dietary supply is needed to stay healthy.

If a 'free radical' attacks a cell it combines with the fatty constituents of that cell to produce lipid (i.e. fatty) peroxides. These lipid peroxides are highly reactive and in their turn generate even more free radicals which eventually destroy the cell. This mechanism of 'free radical' attack is believed to be the cause of many of the degenerative diseases of the body that affect the heart, muscles, vital organs and joints. Cancer is probably a result of uncontrolled cellular oxidation.

PREVENTING THE EFFECTS OF FREE RADICALS

The protective mechanism that stops the harmful effects of free radicals and peroxides is believed to reside in the three anti-oxidants; vitamin E, vitamin C and selenium. Selenium is some 50 to 100 times more active as an anti-oxidant than vitamin E. Vitamin C is just as important as vitamin E as a protective agent and they work together synergistically. Both vitamins are required daily in similar high amounts.

The mode of action of selenium and vitamin E depends upon a specific enzyme called glutathione peroxidase. An enzyme is defined as a living catalyst, that is, it accelerates the body reactions that are the basis of life itself. Without these catalysts, body reactions would be too slow to sustain life. Without enzymes there is no life and without vitamins and minerals, enzymes will not function. Glutathione peroxidase, the protective enzyme will not function without selenium and vitamin E, so that all three are essential for removing free radicals and peroxides as they are formed in the body.

The importance of vitamin E and selenium as dietary nutrients is summed up by Dr Denman Harman, President of the American Ageing Association, who has stated that 'diets designed to minimise random free radical reactions in the body may reasonably be expected to add five to ten or more years of healthy productive life to the lifespan of the average person'.

Other functions attributed solely to vitamin E in the past are now known to also need the presence of the mineral selenium. A combination of vitamin E with selenium has been given a two-year clinical trial on angina patients in Mexico and the Philippines. The results indicated that 92 per cent of the patients so treated had relief from recurring attacks of angina pectoris. The beneficial responses included reduction or elimination of angina attacks, increased vigour and work capacity and improved electro-cardiograms (indication of heart function). There was no evidence of side effects with this treatment.

Vitamin E and selenium together help the body resist infection caused by invading bacteria and viruses. A Russian report by Dr T.F. Berenthein claimed that the combination of nutrients was more effective than either one alone. Selenium itself was less effective; vitamin E alone had no effect. Confirmation of these results came from Colorado State University, USA where Dr J.E. Spallholtz and Dr J.L. Martin reported that the vitamin E/selenium mixture increased the body's production of antibodies to infection some 20 to 30 times more than controls.

INHIBITION OF CANCERS

Science News (February 26th 1976) reports: 'the trace mineral selenium with vitamin E and vitamin C actually inhibits cancers in experimental animals'. Cancers included those of the skin, lungs, breast, stomach and liver. They were induced by chemical agents and the combined antioxidants reduced their incidence in animals from 90 per cent to less than 10 per cent.

In human beings, the prime cause of skin cancer is excessive exposure to the ultra-violet rays of sunlight. Dr S. Wan-Bang Lo and S. Black of the Baylor College of Medicine, USA have found that therapy using the antioxidants selenium and vitamins A and C protect against sun-induced cancer. It is apparent that whether cancer is produced by free radicals, chemical agents, or ultra violet light, this combination of nutrients exerts a protective effect.

THE USE OF SELENIUM

In view of this recent research into selenium, it is tempting to postulate that where massive doses of vitamin E have a beneficial effect, the vitamin is covering for a selenium deficiency – which could be the real problem. Tocopherols protect selenium. Conversely, when vitamin E therapy fails, a combined treatment with selenium could be successful.

Selenium/vitamin E treatment has been used for many years in veterinary practice for helping animals with arthritis and muscular dystrophy. Dr Wilfred Shute, the pioneer of vitamin E therapy believes that selenium could be beneficial in some vitamin E – resistant cases and he calls for controlled clinical trials in this respect. He agrees that the mineral will probably reduce the need for the vitamin and this combination is more likely to be effective than either nutrient alone.

THE ANTAGONISTS OF VITAMIN E

Any constituent that inhibits the action of vitamin E either in body processes or in the diet is known as an antagonist. The most widely studied antagonists that are essential to body processes are the female sex hormones called oestrogens. Iron is believed to be the most important antagonist to the vitamin when administered as an oral supplement.

OESTROGENS AND VITAMIN E

There is now direct evidence that the administration

of oestrogens has a deleterious effect upon the vitamin E status of the body. Oestrogens are given for a variety of complaints but often the treatment is short-term and any effect upon other body constituents is purely temporary. However, there are two uses where oestrogens are given for prolonged periods and these are in contraception and during the menopause.

Most contraceptive pills contain synthetic oestrogens that are more potent on a weight-for-weight basis than those occurring naturally. These synthetic oestrogens appear to exert a direct inhibiting action on vitamin E. The blood levels of the vitamin tend to be low in women on the pill due to direct inhibition of absorption of the vitamin and excessive destruction within the body.

In a report to the American College of Physicians, Doctors Weinberger, Collins and Luetscher of the Stanford University School of Medicine stated that high blood pressure developed in women who had been taking 'the pill' for as little as one year. Even after refraining from taking 'the pill' only 50 per cent of those affected had their blood pressure return to normal after a period of 6 months. A national study in the USA termed the *Coronary Drug Project* concluded that after 5 years on this oestrogenic treatment, an excessive number of women experienced heart attacks, lung disease and blood clots in the circulatory system.

A report in the medical journal *M.D.* of Canada in October 1973 noted that a similar study on a large number of women revealed eleven times the incidence of thrombosis and double the incidence of gall bladder disease when compared with women not on the pill. All of these effects upon the heart and blood system are related to the antagonistic property of oestrogens against vitamin E, according to the researchers involved.

Treatment of the menopause with oestrogens is not generally accepted in the UK but it is widespread on the continent of Europe. *The Medical Post* for 20th February 1973 reported that there was no evidence that routine treatment with oestrogens helped the emotional symptoms of the menopause. Nor were there any beneficial effects upon other symptoms associated with the condition.

After a lifetime of experience, doctors Evan Shute and Wilfred Shute, both obstetricians and gynaecologists, have found a better response in the menopause to alpha tocopherol. They believe that giving oestrogens merely reduced the tocopherol level in the female and the dangers associated with the hormonal treatment (such as development of cancer) are attributed in part at least to lack of vitamin E.

IRON AND VITAMIN E

It is often stated that in the diet, iron and vitamin E should not be taken together as supplements because iron destroys the vitamin; what is not always realized is that iron exists in two forms, known as ferric and ferrous. Ferric iron destroys vitamin E; ferrous iron does not. This problem was studied by myself when I was engaged on research into the treatment of kidney disease with vitamin E at Liverpool University. It was shown quite conclusively that iron, when presented as ferrous salts in supplements, has no effect on the vitamin E, either outside or inside the body. Iron must be in the ferrous form to be absorbed, which is why supplements are usually in the ferrous form.

In white flour, iron is added because the law

demands it, but usually as ferric salts. Many studies have indicated the uselessness of this fortification because absorption of the iron is negligible. At the same time, the ferric iron can destroy what little vitamin E is left. Any preparation containing ferrous salts such as ferrous sulphate, ferrous chloride or ferrous gluconate with vitamin E is, in the main, quite acceptable. However, the safest way to take iron with the vitamin is as the amino acid, chelate. This is the natural iron as found in food and because it is protected by the amino acids there is no possibility of conversion to ferric iron by other food constituents. This conversion is possible with simple iron salts.

CHAPTER FOUR

NATURAL SOURCES OF VITAMIN E

The tocopherols are widely distributed in nature but their content in foodstuffs varies tremendously. Vitamin E is always present in the natural state as the free tocopherols. This means that they are not combined with acids like acetic and succinic. The richest sources are cereal grain oils like corn (i.e. maize) oil and wheat germ oil. Not all vegetable oils are good sources of the vitamin.

THE VITAMIN E CONTENT OF VEGETABLE OILS

A study has been carried out on vegetable oils by Drs D.C. Herting and E.E. Drury at the laboratories of Distillation Products Industries of New York, one of the world's largest producers of vitamin E. It was found that the content of the total tocopherols ranged from 0.2mg per 100g in some samples of coconut oil to almost 200mg per 100g in wheat germ oil. Coconut, olive and linseed oils were found to be practically devoid of the vitamin.

Even in individual types of cereal grains, the tocopherol levels of the extracted oils were found to be influenced by the source of the plant, the time of harvest, the storage conditions and the way in which the cereals were refined. For example, the levels in corn oil varied from 29.5 to 63.6mg per 100g oil and those in soya bean oil from 60.5 to 91.8mg per 100g oil. Table 2 shows the average vitamin E content of various vegetable oils, together with the percentages of the total present as d-alpha tocopherol.

Table 2: Tocopherol contents of various vegetable oils

Source of oil	Total tocopherols mg per 100g oil	Percentage of total present as d-alpha tocopherol
Castor Bean	29.1	0
Cocoa butter	15.5	17.0
Coconut	1.1	45.5
Corn	66.1	15.3
Cottonseed	63.5	50.1
Grapeseed	19.4	77.0
Linseed	6.1	0
Mustard-seed	44.6	31.0
Olive	4.6	100.0
Peanut	21.5	35.6
Rapeseed	43.3	31.9
Rice bran	44.4	59.0
Safflower	49.2	48.3
Soyabean	87.1	10.5
Sunflower	27.1	89.2
Tung	81.0	30.0
Wheat Germ	189.7	71.5

The table illustrates the wide variation in the percentage of d-alpha tocopherol in the total vitamin E present. As present-day knowledge suggests that this type of tocopherol is the most potent biologically, it is important to realize that some vegetable oils are not necessarily good sources of it. On the other hand, a varied diet would be expected to supply all of the four types of vitamin E and it is possible that in some of its functions, tocopherols other than d-alpha are more active. One example is in its protective anti-oxidant action where d-delta tocopherol has been shown to be the most potent.

When seeking a balanced, good quality diet, it is safer to ensure that the vitamin E intake includes all

of the four types prevalent in food. If the vitamin is
being taken in high concentration, as in the case of
medical treatment, however, the d-alpha tocopherol
is the preferred type. Table 3 summarizes the
percentages of the various tocopherols in the
commonly used vegetable oils. The content of d-
gamma tocopherol includes that of d-beta
tocopherol, since these two are impossible to
separate in the methods used for analysis.

The soft margarines that are manufactured from
blended vegetable oils have a reasonable content of
tocopherol but because of the processing method
involved, much of the vitamin is lost. The level in
these margarines is only 8.0mg tocopherol per 100
which is somewhat less than the original levels in the
vegetable oils used to make them.

**Table 3: The Percentages of Various Tocopherols in
Vegetable Oils**

Oils	d-alpha tocopherol	d-beta plus d-gamma tocopherols	d-delta tocopherol
Coconut	45.5	0	54.5
Cottonseed	50.1	49.9	0
Maize	15.3	82.2	2.5
Olive	100.0	0	0
Palm	39.9	49.2	10.9
Peanut	35.6	58.6	5.8
Rapeseed	31.9	66.0	2.1
Safflowerseed	48.3	21.7	30.0
Soyabean	10.5	61.9	27.6
Sunflowerseed	89.2	9.3	1.5
Wheat Germ	71.5	14.0	14.5

LOSS DURING CEREAL PROCESSING
Natural grains often contain appreciable quantities
of vitamin E. The average d-alpha tocopherol

contents of whole corn, wheat, oats and rice are 1.53, 0.87, 1.54 and 0.26mg per 100g respectively. These values can vary up to three-fold, however, when measured in various samples. This is because of the variability of such factors as strain of plant, the area where the grain is grown, the time of harvest and storage conditions after harvest.

A comprehensive study comparing cereal grains and processed cereals published in the journal *Agriculture and Food Chemistry* in 1969 reported that virtually any type of processing of whole cereal grains results in losses of the vitamin E content.

In the case of corn, loss ranged from 35 per cent when it was made into white meal to 98 per cent when the grain was converted into corn flakes. Puffed wheat has 22 per cent less d-alpha tocopherol than the original grain. Producing white flour from wheat grain causes 92 per cent of the original tocopherol to be lost. Simple production of oatmeal results in little or no decrease in the vitamin E content. More extensive processing of oats to produce highly refined flakes increased loss of the vitamin to 95 per cent. Whenever rice was processed in any form, losses of vitamin E were consistently above 70 per cent.

METHODS OF PROCESSING

The variability of vitamin E losses lies in the methods of processing. Oatmeal shows little reduction in level because only the hull is removed and the processing is mild. Cornmeal, on the other hand, is made by removing both the hull and most of the germ, which is rich in tocopherol, so that the product as eaten contains little tocopherol.

Some cereals are more highly refined and removal of parts of the grain followed by flaking, shredding, or puffing results in serious losses of the vitamin.

Oddly, the production of puffed wheat from the grain causes little reduction in the vitamin E content but a similar process to produce puffed rice reduces the content by 40 per cent. When brown rice is milled the bran fraction is removed, taking most of the vitamin with it. Parboiling of the resultant white rice induces further losses. The production of white flour (74 per cent extraction) from wheat leads to 92 per cent loss of the original d-alpha tocopherol content.

The effects of processing on the d-alpha tocopherol content of grains are summarized in Table 4. The results emphasize the superiority of eating cereals in the whole grain, unprocessed form, compared to the highly refined cereals that today represent the most popular way to eat these important food products.

The highest intake of grain in most modern diets is in the form of wheat flour that has been baked into bread. There are striking differences between the vitamin E content of white and wholemeal bread. The total tocopherols in white bread are only 0.23mg per 100g bread compared with 2.2mg per 100g of wholemeal bread.

This staggering loss of 90 per cent of the vitamin E is due to two factors. First, much of the wheat germ which is the source of vitamin E is removed during the production of white flour. Second, the most common flour 'improver' in producing white bread is a compound called chlorine dioxide, which is known to destroy vitamin E. The tragedy is that although the manufacture of white bread is known to cause wholesale loss of vitamin E, there is no law that says it must be put back. The person who eats 8 slices of white bread per day (300g) is receiving only 0.69mg vitamin E as opposed to the 6.6mg they would receive from the same intake of wholemeal bread.

Table 4: The effect of processing on the vitamin E content of cereal grains

Grain	Processed form	d-alpha tocopherol mg per 100g	percentage loss
Corn	Whole Grain	1.53	
	Meal	0.42	73
	Grits	0.35	77
	Flakes	0.08	95
	Puffed	0.09	94
	Shredded	0.08	95
Wheat	Whole Grain	0.87	
	Meal	0.11	87
	Flour	0.07	92
	Flakes	0.25	71
	Puffed	0.68	22
	Shredded	0.09	90
Oats	Whole Grains	1.54	
	Stored 6 years	0.42	73
	Rolled	1.33	14
	Shredded	0.08	95
	Granular	0.08	95
Rice	Whole Grain	0.35	
	Parboiled	0.15	57
	Dehulled brown	0.26	26
	Dehulled parboiled	0.15	57
	Milled white	0.10	71
	Milled parboiled	0.06	83
	Expanded	0.01	97
	Puffed	0.07	80
	Shredded	0.02	94
	Meal	0.10	71

VITAMIN E LOSS DURING FOOD PROCESSING

Fruit and vegetables do not contribute significant amounts of d-alpha tocopherol to the diet. The preservation of vegetables such as peas leads to substantial losses of the vitamin regardless of the method used. Fresh, frozen and tinned peas contain respectively 1.73, 0.65 and 0.04mg total tocopherols per 100g peas. The d-alpha tocopherol content is respectively 0.55, 0.25 and 0.02mg per 100g peas.

Home cooking of vegetables when confined to boiling or steaming for 30 minutes reduces the tocopherol content by only 3.7 per cent. Commercial processing and storage, however, lead to considerable losses of the vitamin. Deep fat frying represents much more serious reduction in the vitamin E levels of foods. The oil used for frying loses little of its tocopherol (usually about 11 per cent) but the foods that have been fried, such as potato crisps and chips, lose a substantial portion of their vitamin E, even at low temperature storage.

For instance it was found that potato crips lose 48 per cent of their vitamin E after only two weeks at room temperature. After two months under these conditions this loss had increased to 77 per cent. When stored at deep freeze temperatures of -12°C, vitamin E losses still totalled 68 per cent after two months. French fried potatoes that were stored at this low temperature lost 68 per cent and 74 per cent of their vitamin E after storage periods of one month and two months respectively.

FROZEN FOODS AND VEGETABLE OILS
This loss of tocopherol in frozen foods is of considerable importance today, because of the increasing consumption of foods of this type. The simplest way to maintain the vitamin E level in fried frozen foods of any type is to fortify the vegetable oils used in their preparation with d-alpha tocopheryl acetate. It was shown in Chapter One that this form

of vitamin E is far more stable than d-alpha tocopherol itself, when in contact with high temperatures and air.

However, there is no way of knowing if a commercial producer of frozen foods has supplemented his products with vitamin E unless this is stated on the label. The individual who cooks with vegetable oils has a much greater control over the type of oil used and is able to choose the most suitable one.

Vegetable oils are obtained from the grains in either of two ways. In the first, the grain is crushed under high pressure and the oil is literally squeezed from it at ordinary room temperatures. The product is known as a cold-pressed oil. There is no destruction of the vitamin E with this process, it is retained in the finished product.

The second and cheaper way of extracting oils is to treat the crushed grain with a solvent that will dissolve the oils present. The solvent containing the oils is then clarified by filtration and heated to remove the solvent, leaving the oil as residue. This process reduces the vitamin E content considerably. Some manufacturers then add the vitamin as d-alpha tocopheryl acetate to restore the material that was lost.

Hence the safest measure to ensure that the vegetable oil that you use is adequate in vitamin E is either to use a cold-pressed oil or ensure that your brand has added vitamin E. This will be stated on the label.

OTHER FOODS

Animal fats are generally poor sources of vitamin E compared to vegetable oils and fats. Cod liver oil is very rich in the vitamin but as it does not feature in any great quantity in most daily diets, this source is of less importance. Although meats are not especially rich in the vitamin, they do contain a high proportion of their vitamin E content as d-alpha tocopherol. Beef liver contains the highest level amongst the meats.

Dairy products are not particularly rich in vitamin E, with the exception of eggs. Two eggs supply 2.4mg of tocopherols and all the vitamin is located in the yolk. It is significant that the milk from cows on pastures is four times richer in vitamin E than that from stall-fed animals.

Fresh fruits do not contribute very much tocopherol to the diet but in all fruits studied, over 90 per cent of the tocopherol present is there as the d-alpha tocopherol form. Fresh vegetables also tend to be low in the vitamin, with sweet potato and turnip green contributing the highest amounts. The proportion of d-alpha tocopherol is variable but on the whole this isomer predominates in vegetables.

The total tocopherol content of various foods is given in Table 5. The amount of these tocopherols present as d-alpha has also been tabulated.

THE AVERAGE DAILY INTAKE OF D-ALPHA TOCOPHEROL

No one is certain exactly how much vitamin E needs to be taken in the diet each day to maintain health, although it is generally accepted that the requirements increase with an increased intake of polyunsaturated fatty acids (from vegetable oils).

A review of the problem was published by the British Nutrition Foundation in May 1975. In this it was stated that 'it was likely that in many relatively affluent countries the average daily intake of vitamin E does not approach the recommended values'. Typical American diets contain only 8.2 to 23.7 i.u. of biologically available vitamin E with a mean of

Table 5: Tocopherol Content of Foods

Food	Total Tocopherols (mg per 100g)	d-alpha Tocopherol (mg per 100g)
Fresh Fruits:		
Apples	0.51	0.31
Bananas	0.42	0.22
Strawberries	0.40	0.21
Melon	0.31	0.14
Grapefruit	0.25	0.21
Oranges	0.23	0.22
Orange Juice	0.20	0.04
Canned Tomato Juice	0.71	0.22
Canned Grapefruit Juice	0.18	0.04
Vegetables:		
Crisps	11.40	6.40
Fried Onion Rings	6.40	0.65
Sweet Potato	4.00	4.00
Turnip Greens	2.24	2.19
Fresh Peas	1.73	0.55
Fresh Green Beans	1.68	0.47
French Fried Potatoes Brand B	1.59	0.43
Baked Beans	1.16	0.14

Tomatoes	0.85	0.40
Frozen Peas – Cooked	0.65	0.25
Frozen Peas – Uncooked	0.64	0.22
Celery	0.57	0.38
French Fried Potatoes Brand A	0.36	0.12
Yellow Onion	0.34	0.22
Frozen Cut Green Beans – Cooked	0.25	0.11
Frozen Cut Green Beans – Uncooked	0.24	0.09
Carrots	0.21	0.11
Lettuce	0.17	0.06
Raw Potato	0.085	0.053
Boiled Potato	0.061	0.043
Baked Potato	0.055	0.027
Canned Green Beans	0.05	0.03
Canned Peas	0.04	0.02
Cereals:		
Oatmeal	3.23	2.27
Muesli	3.20	1.72
Brown Rice	2.40	1.20
All-Bran	2.00	2.27
Weetabix	1.80	0.87
Puffed Wheat	1.70	0.85

continued overleaf

Table 5 (cont)

Food	Total Tocopherols (mg per 100g)	d-alpha Tocopherol (mg per 100g)
Grapenuts	1.60	0.77
Ready Brek	1.20	0.62
Shredded Wheat	1.00	0.52
Polished Rice	0.62	0.35
Rice Krispies	0.60	0.31
Special K	0.50	0.22
Cornflakes	0.40	0.22
Cooked White Rice	0.27	0.18
Wholemeal Bread	2.20	0.45
White Bread	0.23	0.10
Cooked Meats:		
Broiled Beef Liver	1.62	0.63
Roast Frozen Chicken	1.39	0.44
Corned Beef	0.78	0.44
Liver Sausage	0.69	0.35
Roast Beef	0.63	0.37
Roast Pork	0.60	0.16
Fried Bacon	0.59	0.53
Broiled Chicken	0.58	0.37

Fried Ham Steak	0.52	0.28
Fried Pork Sausage	0.32	0.16
Roast Lamb	0.32	0.16
Roast Veal	0.24	0.05
Dairy Products:		
Egg Yolk	4.60	1.58
Whole Egg	1.63	0.56
Butter	1.0	1.0
Whole Milk	0.093	0.036
Egg White	0	0
Other Products:		
Cod Liver Oil	20.00	18.12
Dry Roasted Peanuts	11.70	7.70
Mayonnaise	9.00	6.00
Margarine	8.00	6.38
Peanut Butter	7.67	6.00
Shrimps	6.60	0.61
Salmon Steak	1.81	1.35
Suet	1.50	0.92
Haddock Fillet	1.20	0.60
Beef Dripping	0.3	0.2
Lard	Trace	Trace

16.8 i.u. Both Canadian and British diets contain considerably less than the recommended intake of vitamin E.

The most recent recommended daily allowance of vitamin E by US authorities was in September 1977. They suggest an absolute minimum of 15 i.u. vitamin E but prefer a level of 30 i.u. for adults per day. According to the same source, pregnant and lactating women should take between 30 and 60 i.u. per day. They do not recommend any upper limits for adults because of the lack of toxicity of vitamin E. UK official Government Authorities are unwilling to suggest a daily requirement but claim that most diets provide at least 10 i.u. of vitamin E per day but do not specify which type of vitamin this figure refers to.

Typical diets for Europe and the United States have been calculated to contain only about 15mg (i.e. 21.2 i.u.) of d-alpha tocopherol per day. Table 6 gives the quantities of vitamin E likely to be provided in the usual Western diets.

Although this figure is above the minimum quantity recommended by the US Government, it falls far short of the 30 i.u. per day that they prefer as a daily intake.

An International Symposium on Vitamin E held in Minneapolis during September 1977 made the following recommendations about vitamin E supplementation. Large amounts of tocopherol must be eaten in order to induce small rises in the blood level. For example, to double the blood content it is essential to increase the daily vitamin E intake 40-fold. This means that an individual who is receiving a minimum of 10 i.u. per day from the diet would have to take a supplement of 400 i.u. daily to increase their blood levels two-fold. There is no way that 400

Typical Daily Intake of Vitamin E

Food	Daily Consumption in grams	d-alpha tocopherol intake in i.u.
Fats and Oils (with butter)	81	11.7
Grain Products	213	2.7
Meat, Poultry, Fish	196	1.5
Potatoes	143	1.3
Eggs	58	1.0
Dairy Products (without butter)	536	0.9
Green Vegetables	142	0.7
Dried peas, beans, nuts	20	0.6
Citrus fruits and tomatoes	131	0.5
Other fruits and vegetables	29	0.2
Coffee, tea and other beverages	24	0.1
Sugar	132	0.0
		21.2

i.u. could be obtained from the diet alone, so supplementation is essential.

A daily supplement of 100 i.u. of the vitamin will give reasonable blood levels but increasing this to 500 i.u. per day will only increase the blood tocopherol by 10 per cent. In other words, the higher the blood level, the more difficult it is to increase it. For these reasons, to increase the intake gradually over a period of time is a more economical way to raise body vitamin E levels than to take a high concentration immediately.

The absorption and assimilation of tocopherols in healthy people is considerably less than 100 per cent. This figure is reduced even more in those who, for one reason or another, are unable to absorb fats and oils fully. Although 70 per cent of a low intake of vitamin E (i.e. up to 100 i.u. per day) is absorbed, less is utilized in the body as the intake increases. These figures all refer to d-alpha tocopherol oils. The amount absorbed is much higher when the vitamin is presented in the water-solubilized form.

The relatively poor efficiency of absorption of vitamin E means that very high concentrations must be taken when the vitamin is being used to treat certain diseases. Doses of 3,500 i.u. per day are not uncommon in the treatment of heart and blood circulation complaints. Such doses are essential to raise the blood and tissue levels to concentrations that can do some good. Because these intakes are so high, it is essential for such treatment to be under medical supervision. No one should attempt to take them without clinical monitoring of their condition. The highest potency that can be taken by most people in safety is 1,000 i.u. per day either, in a single dose or spread over 24 hours.

CHAPTER FIVE

SOME CONDITIONS THAT HAVE BEEN HELPED BY VITAMIN E

The usefulness of vitamin E in treating many illnesses is still a controversial subject among contemporary doctors. The main proponents of the vitamin as a therapeutic agent remain the medical staff of the Shute Foundation for Medical Research in Canada. However, a search of the medical literature indicates that there are now many other clinical groups around the world who have reported the beneficial effects from vitamin E in various diseases, with and without the more medically accepted drugs.

Equally so, many doctors have been unable to detect any response to treatment with the vitamins. It must be stated, however, that differences in opinion of its efficacy often relate to variations in dosage, length of time of treatment and selection of patients. Vitamin E may also have a protective effect against many clinical conditions but it is always more difficult to prove prevention than observe a beneficial effect upon an existing condition.

The main groups of diseases that have responded to vitamin E are essentially those of the blood circulation system, where for one reason or another, the flow of blood to an organ or muscle has been curtailed. This may be due to a blood clot (thrombosis); a narrowing of the blood vessel due to deposition of fat (atherosclerosis); a hardening of the artery (arteriosclerosis); a swollen and knotted condition of the veins (varicose veins); blood clots in the veins (thrombophlebitis); abnormal blood capillary permeability in the kidney (nephritis).

Other conditions include high blood-pressure, rheumatic fever, heart failure, sterility, menstrual problems and ageing. In addition, some skin diseases – including severe ulceration – have been reported to respond to vitamin E treatment.

(i) *Intermittent Claudication*

This is the term that describes the cramping pain in the calf muscles that is produced on exercise. It is caused by a narrowing of the arteries supplying blood to the leg muscles. The restricted blood supply gives rise to the pain as the muscles become starved of oxygen. There are at least 35 publications in the Western world medical press confirming the excellent reponse of this condition to d-alpha tocopherol. A leading article in *The Lancet* in 1974 states that this is the only generally accepted use of vitamin E in medical practice.

In 1958 Dr P.D. Livingstone and Dr C. Jones reported the results of a double-blind clinical trial of vitamin E in intermittent claudication carried out at Sheffield. A double-blind trial compares the effect of the vitamin with a harmless compound (placebo) in a similar presentation in the treatment of the condition. Double-blind simply means that neither patient nor doctor knows which is which until the end of the trial. In this way the result cannot be influenced by personal bias.

Out of 17 patients who were treated with 600 i.u. of d-alpha tocopherol per day for a total period of 40 weeks, 13 showed significant improvement in their ability to walk without pain. Only 2 of the 17 patients treated with the placebo reported some improvement over a similar period. One important feature to arise was that it was essential to continue treatment for at least 3 months before any improvement became apparent. At the same time it was noted that the vitamin E-treated patients had an increased life survival rate. Eventually this research group was able to report in 1963 that some 1,500 patients suffering from intermittent claudication had responded favourably and significantly to tocopherol treatment.

FURTHER VITAMIN E TESTS

A more recent study was carried out in Sweden and reported in 1974 by Dr Knut Haeger. This group of patients suffered from intermittent claudication during periods ranging from 4 to 7 years. A total of 81 patients were treated with conventional medicinal drugs. An additional 44 were treated with a multi-vitamin preparation but since there was no response they were switched to vitamin E alone. A total of 104 patients received vitamin E alone from the start, at an initial dose of 600 i.u. per day reducing to 300 i.u.

All patients in the study were treated for 2 years but 69.2 per cent continued treatment for 3 years or more. There were twice as many deaths in the groups not receiving vitamin E. Four times as many patients on vitamin E as those not treated with it were able to increase their walking distance. Ten times as many of those receiving the vitamin as the untreated ones were able to more than double their walking distances without experiencing pain.

When intermittent claudication does not respond to treatment, the condition may eventually lead to amputation of the afflicted limb. In Dr Haeger's study the number of amputations in the control group to those receiving vitamin E was 11:1. All of these figures represent a significant improvement in those suffering from intermittent claudication who were treated with vitamin E.

Modern thinking suggests that patients suffering from intermittent claudication should be forced into regular walking exercises to the utmost extent possible. This, together with a daily dose of vitamin E up to 1200 i.u. per day, can help virtually every patient. Recent studies indicate that between 2g and 5g of vitamin C should also be taken to help relieve the constricted blood flow. Vitamin E helps in this disease because it decreases the oxygen requirements of the affected muscles; it prevents the formation of a thrombus or blood clot and it speeds up the development of alternative blood supplies to the muscles.

(ii) *Angina Pectoris*

Angina pectoris is a condition characterized by a severe, constricting pain in the chest, usually radiating to one or both arms and shoulders. The pain is due to a temporary insufficiency of blood to the heart that deprives the heart muscle of oxygen. It is a similar situation to that in intermittent claudication, except that the heart muscle itself is affected instead of the legs. In both cases the attack is relieved by rest.

Conventional treatment for angina is aimed at reducing the work load of the heart and widening the blood vessels with drugs in order to increase the blood flow. The treatment only causes temporary relief – it does nothing to overcome the basic cause of the disease, which is simply insufficient oxygen supply to the heart muscle. This fact was demonstrated in 1964 by Dr Lawrence S. Cohen of Harvard Medical School and reported by him to the Thirteenth Annual Convention of the American College of Cardiology in New Orleans.

According to the Shute Institute, where many thousands of angina patients have been treated with vitamin E, the angina condition usually responds in 4 to 6 weeks from the start of the treatment. The initial dose is usually 800 i.u. d-alpha tocopherol per day. If there is no improvement after six weeks on this dose, the daily intake is increased by 200 to 400 i.u. for the next six weeks.

When the dose at which the symptoms are relieved is reached, this is continued permanently. Such doses apply only when the blood-pressure is controlled by drugs. Even if there is not complete relief with this treatment, it is important for anyone suffering from angina to take d-alpha tocopherol to prevent blood clots or thrombosis from forming.

(iii) *Coronary Heart Disease*

The coronary arteries supply blood and hence oxygen to the heart muscle itself, so allowing that organ to function effectively. There are two types of coronary heart disease: (1) that due to partial or total blockage of the artery by a blood clot; and (2) that due to a thickening of the artery wall. Sudden or gradual constriction of a coronary artery is thus a very serious state of affairs. Some of the heart muscle is completely deprived of blood and that area of muscle literally dies. The surrounding area may suffer only a temporary shortage of oxygen but this still has the effect of impairing the activity of the heart muscle.

D-alpha tocopherol helps in the coronary heart disease by: (1) dissolving the blood clot that is causing the obstruction; (2) decreasing the oxygen needs of the whole zone of injury, so preserving its structure and function; (3) dilating the blood vessels, so allowing more blood and hence more oxygen to reach the damaged portion of the heart. Continuous use of tocopherol following a heart attack prevents further occurrence of a blockage. Although the heart muscle that has died (known as an infarct) can never be restored, vitamin E treatment ensures that the surrounding area receives adequate oxygen and helps restore it to health.

Even when vitamin E therapy is started immediately after the heart attack, it may take a week or 10 days before any benefit is felt. A study was carried out on 22 patients by Dr W.M. Toone in 1973 and reported in the New Zealand *Journal of Medicine*. Eleven of his patients received 1600 i.u. of d-alpha tocopherol succinate per day after their heart attacks, while the remaining 11 received a placebo. Seven of the treated patients were able to eliminate conventional medical treatment, and all felt the benefit of vitamin E. Only 3 of the control group were able to reduce their medical treatment.

Other studies of the Shute Institute on many hundreds of patients have indicated an overall success rate of 60 per cent of patients receiving vitamin E after a heart attack. The usual procedure is to start such patients on 800 i.u. of vitamin E per day and increase this by 200 i.u. increments every six weeks until a response is obtained. Once the dosage is established, the individual keeps it at that level for the rest of his life.

(iv) *Arteriosclerosis and Cerebral Thrombosis*
A similar dosage regime is carried out on those whose heart blood vessels are constricted by hardening, a condition usually associated with ageing. When a similar condition affects the brain blood vessels, the usual symptoms are forgetfulness, lack of concentration and impaired mental ability in the aged. In both cases vitamin E may be helpful but the addition of vitamin C at a dose of 2g to 5g per day is now known to be particularly beneficial.

A constriction of the blood supply to the brain

(called cerebral thrombosis) may give rise to a stroke resulting in temporary or permanent paralysis of part of the body. Treatment with vitamin E is essentially the same as that when the heart is similarly affected. Not only does vitamin E help dissolve the obstruction but it prevents further formation of thrombi.

(v) *Thrombophlebitis and Varicose Veins*

When blood clots are formed in the veins, the condition is known as thrombophlebitis. Occasionally such clots break up and the pieces are carried in the blood stream to cause constriction elsewhere. When they stop in the lung, the condition is known as pulmonary embolism and it can be fatal. The most likely time for blood clots to form is during or after surgical operations and during childbirth.

Vitamin E treatment before and after surgery is claimed to be the best way to prevent such blood clots from forming. Usually potent anti-blood clotting drugs are used but these can cause severe side-effects, such as haemorrhage. Vitamin E is safe and has the ability to prevent pre-formed clots from breaking up and is also able to dissolve them. Professor Alton Ochsner has claimed in *Postgraduate Medicine* (1968) that he has had no evidence of pulmonary embolism after surgery since using vitamin E as a countermeasure, both before and after the operation.

There are many confirmatory studies coming from places as far apart as Texas, Sweden and Italy. The important feature in all cases was to continue to keep the patient on vitamin E for a long period after the operation. Although daily doses of 800 i.u. were needed to build up the body level of the vitamin before surgery, these were reduced to 200 i.u. per day for a period of several weeks afterwards in order to keep those people free from blood clotting complications.

A second disease of the blood circulatory system is varicose veins. The conventional medical treatment for this condition is surgery. This may be avoided in some cases by treating with vitamin E but the dosage varies over a wide range. Dr W. Shute in his book *Vitamin E for Ailing and Healthy Hearts* quotes many successful treatments of varicose veins with vitamin E.

The dose usually begins at 150 i.u. or 300 i.u. per day which is increased in increments of 100 i.u. every six weeks if no improvement is noted. Most people respond to 300 or 600 i.u. but some need the high dose of 800 i.u. per day before relief is obtained. One of the complications of varicose veins can be the development of ulcers (called indolent ulcers), that are very resistant to healing. Oral vitamin E has been claimed to cut down the incidence of these.

VITAMIN E IN DIABETES

Diabetes is characterized by an increased blood sugar which reflects the sufferer's inability to control the level of this essential blood nutrient. The hormone insulin and various oral drugs, even strict dietary restriction, can all control the blood sugar level satisfactorily. Unfortunately, in the later stage of diabetes, despite this control of the blood sugar, other conditions develop such as kidney disease, high blood-pressure, heart failure, arteriosclerosis, blindness, neuritis and sometimes gangrene.

Many studies from all over the world have confirmed that adequate vitamin E taken as soon as diabetes is diagnosed can prevent the development of these conditions later on in life. There are cases on record where these manifestations have actually cleared up with vitamin E treatment.

Two such cases are reported with photographic

evidence in the *Canadian Medical Association Journal* of 1957. A diabetic woman of 85 developed gangrene of the left great toe. She was given 600 i.u. of d-alpha tocopherol daily along with insulin and a diet to control the diabetes. After 4 days her tocopherol intake was increased to 1,200 i.u. per day which, after one month, caused the affected area to be isolated, preventing the rest of the foot from becoming gangrenous. This allowed the toe to be removed, leaving a clean healing of the wound left after amputation. At the same time it was noted that her insulin requirement dropped dramatically while on vitamin E treatment.

A woman who had been diabetic for 33 years developed gangrene of the right heel. On 1,200 i.u. of vitamin E per day her insulin requirement dropped to a quarter of that previously. At the end of $4\frac{1}{2}$ months the area of gangrene had been neatly separated and there was no spread of the condition. The remainder of the heel cleared up completely to give a clean area that did not contract. The result was that the patient was able to walk in comfort with only a pressure pad in her shoe. Her insulin requirement was stabilized at the new lower level.

Many such cases have been quoted in the medical literature. The best preventive dose for any diabetic, according to the Shute Foundation for Medical Research, is 400 i.u. per day. Once the blood circulation changes have set in however, higher doses – as in the above examples – may be needed.

It is important that any diabetic who wishes to take vitamin E in high dose should do so under medical supervision. This is essential because in one-third of diabetics so treated, insulin dosage needs to be decreased. Only blood sugar monitoring can decide by how much in order to keep the level at normal concentration.

FERTILITY AND VIRILITY

According to Dr Evan Shute writing in *Urological and Cutaneous Reviews*, lack of vitamin E leads to wasting of the reproductive parts in men, first resulting in the inability to produce sperm, followed by complete sterility. He reported a high success rate of extended and prolonged virility/fertility with extra vitamin E intake. Dr E. Lindner in the *International Z. Vitaminforsch* claimed he was able to increase the sperm count of men unable to produce normal spermatozoa. He gave them a daily dose of between 150 and 200 i.u. of vitamin E orally for periods ranging from 8 to 10 weeks and demonstrated an increase in their reproductive ability. Normal sperm count values were achieved in 20 men and a further 21 showed improvement. Of the 20, 17 eventually became virile and fertile.

Sperm counts were boosted dramatically in men given 30 i.u. of d-alpha tocopherol twice per day in a study reported by Dr J.W. Milten in *Nutritional Bases of Reproduction*. Increased density of spermatozoa in their semen was found in 23 out of 50 patients treated. A further 17 responded to the vitamin with an increased volume of seminal fluid. All 40 successfully treated men had greater strength and movement in their sperm, so that the quality of their reproductive process was increased. This resulted in a higher fertility rate amonst these men.

Unfortunately, d-alpha tocopherol appears to have no effect on the sterility of human females. What it does, however, is to prevent miscarriages in those who can conceive but cannot give birth. A comprehensive study of vitamin E in 100 cases was reported by Dr Bayer of West Germany in the journal *Wein. Med. Wochschr*. Half of the couples were troubled with primary infertility, i.e. they were able to conceive but miscarriages were always the result. Out of 144 pregnancies, all were lost. The males were supplemented with 100 i.u. of vitamin E per day and the females were given 200 i.u. per day for 3 months prior to conception. The result was 79 pregnancies, of which only 2 were lost. The abortion rate dropped from 100 per cent to 2.5 per cent.

The second group were classed as secondary infertility, which means that out of 101 pregnancies there were only 38 births. A similar vitamin supplementation régime as before was carried out. The result was a 100 per cent success with 41 pregnancies coming to term, with 41 successful deliveries. Any dosage less than this produced a decreased rate of success.

MENSTRUAL PROBLEMS

The use of vitamin E in the menopause has been actively studied by Dr Henry A. Gozan of New York. In the *New York State Journal of Medicine* he reported that treatment with vitamin E helped relieve the flushing, headaches and nervous symptoms associated with the menopause. There was success in easing and eliminating these distressing symptoms in 59 out of 66 patients so treated. The dosage used was 100 i.u. of the vitamin taken 3 times daily over a 3 month period.

There are many reports of the beneficial effects of vitamin E in relieving the painful periods suffered by some women and in normalizing the cycle where this is irregular. Heavy and scanty menstrual flows are not influenced by the vitamin.

According to the Shute Institute, vitamin E exerts its action in females by normalizing the blood levels of the female sex hormones, known as oestrogens. It dilates the blood vessels, so ensuring a good supply of blood to the womb. At the same time, the vitamin improves the heat-regulating capacity of the body,

which is why it helps in the excessive sweating that is
often a feature of the menopause.

Menstrual abnormalities are often treated with
oestrogens. However, many obstetricians and
gynaecologists who have used vitamin E believe it is
safer to let the vitamin stimulate the body's own
production of oestrogens. There is a certain risk in
treating females with sex hormones, particularly
during the menopause, when their production starts
to slow down. By treating with vitamin E it is
believed that the transition to decreased production
of oestrogens, with its accompanying effects, is
smoother and easier. Similarly, irregular oestrogen
synthesis which can give rise to problems in the
younger females may be normalized by vitamin E
treatment.

HOW VITAMIN E MAY BE USED ON THE SKIN

Whenever the skin is damaged by accident or
disease, the prime requirement for the healing
process is an ample supply of oxygen. This is
provided in the modern treatment of large scale
burns by literally suspending the patient in a stream
of sterile oxygen by means of specially constructed
beds. The technique has been proved to cause faster
healing and reduced scar formation. Vitamin E
is able to perform a similar function by stimulating
the supply of oxygen to the damaged skin. This it
does by a two-pronged approach. First, it is applied
to the skin in an ointment or cream. Second, it is
taken orally to help the healing process from inside
the body.

SUNBURN

The effectiveness of vitamin E in treating burns from
whatever cause is proved in 30 published medical

reports in medical journals from all parts of the
world. Sunburn is one condition that responds
particularly well to vitamin E ointment. A girl
suffering from intense sunburn over most of her body
was liberally covered with vitamin E ointment.
Although, for various reasons, this was delayed for
20 hours after exposure, after an hour of treatment
she recovered completely – with no signs of blisters
or peeling.

A man suffered very bad sunburn over the whole of
his back. In an attempt to test the effectiveness of
vitamin E ointment, this was used to cover half the
sunburnt area. The other half was left untreated.
The following day there was no sign of sunburn on
the treated half but in complete contrast, the area left
alone was covered in large blisters. These took a
week to heal. Fortunately, photographs were taken
and the case was used to illustrate the healing power
of vitamin E applied topically (i.e. on the skin) to a
Medical Congress in California.

SCALDING

When the skin is damaged by scalds or hot objects
the results are far more serious than simple sunburn,
yet vitamin E is just as effective. Dr Wilfred E. Shute
reports two very serious cases of scalding in his book
Vitamin E for Ailing and Healthy Hearts. A boy of six
was scalded badly with multiple burns over his neck,
torso, back, chest and thigh. An attempt at skin-
grafting was not only unsuccessful but left whole
areas of raw flesh that were badly infected. This
persisted for 10 weeks. Treatment with vitamin E
was then initiated. After 10 days, the infection was
cleared but the damaged areas remained very raw
and painful. Application of vitamin E ointment was
continued, along with a daily oral dose of 300 i.u.
Complete healing occurred after 13 weeks. What

was particularly gratifying was to find that the scars
were smooth, painless and not contracted into
wheals. Skin-grafting was not even needed.

Older people respond just as dramatically. A
woman aged 58 received scalds over a wide area of
her torso and the damage was worsened by leaving
on her clothing, which retained the hot water next to
the skin. Conventional medical treatment with brine
baths failed, leaving her with a grossly infected skin.
Treatment was switched to oral and topical vitamin
E. Within 5 days healing commenced and
continuation of the treatment for 3 months resulted
in complete cure.

Dr Wilfred E. Shute attributes the healing
properties of vitamin E on the skin to three unique
characteristics: (1) it lessens or removes the
associated pain a few minutes after application; (2)
it stops the burn from deepening, limiting the
damage to the cells actually destroyed by the
burning agent; (3) it stimulates rapid regeneration
of new skin, giving a scar that is not painful, is of the
same height as surrounding skin and is not
contracted.

The mild antiseptic quality of vitamin E may help
against infection but other measures are usually
needed to keep the affected area clean. Once this is
controlled, the healing action of the vitamin is both
quick and effective.

LEG ULCERS AND OTHER SKIN CONDITIONS

Some leg ulcers are very resistant to conventional
medical treatment and they often persist for long
periods. They are prone to infection and cause a
severe, burning and aching pain. Despite some 60
publications in medical journals of the effectiveness
of vitamin E ointment for treating them, these ulcers

are still a big problem for many people. They are associated with a poor blood supply to the limb, caused usually by varicose veins.

Application of the ointment and oral supplementation of the vitamin in the diet are usually sufficient to heal these ulcers. There is a word of caution from the proponents of this treatment, however. Once the ulcer has gone, oral supplementation of vitamin E should continue. This maintains local tissue oxygenation and blood circulation and prevents the ulcers from recurring.

Skin conditions, like acne and eczema, have responded to topical treatment with vitamin E ointment. There are many cases on record where multiple lacerations to the face as received in car accidents are completely and clearly healed up with combined topical and oral vitamin E treatment. Many surgery units now use vitamin E ointment routinely after operations. It reduces toxic reactions, then soothes and heals the irritated areas.

NERVE, JOINT AND MUSCULAR COMPLAINTS

The discovery that tocopherol in ointment form appears to penetrate intact skin has stimulated its trial in nerve, joint and muscular complaints. Doctors Burgess and Pritchard, of the Montreal General Hospital, used the ointment to treat nerve root pain. This is associated with neuritis, neuralgia, sciatica and various cases of muscle inflammation (myositis), including the condition known as frozen shoulder. The ointment was rubbed into the affected area, which was then warmed by external heat to ensure the vitamin reached the roots of the nerves. Most cases responded but when no relief was obtained after 7 days, the treatment was felt unlikely to help.

Similar trials on patients suffering from rheumatoid arthritis were reported from The Shute Institute. Vitamin E ointment brought about a reduction of swelling and pain in the joints and there was an increase in mobility. It was found to be extremely effective when rubbed into fingers that were arthritic. The ointment can be of real value in relieving the itching of abdominal skin when this is due to striae, the stretch marks often left after pregnancy or steroid treatment. In the long term treatment, such lesions are often removed completely. Itching associated with the vagina and anus has also been reported to be alleviated with vitamin E ointment.

It is generally agreed amongst the doctors who recommend it that the best potency for vitamin E ointment is 30 i.u. of d-alpha tocopherol per gram of ointment. There have been reports of allergic reactions to this strength of vitamin E when applied to the skin. According to Doctors R.H. Brodkin and J. Bleiberg writing in *Archives of Dermatology*, some 10 per cent of people cannot tolerate this ointment. In these cases diluting the ointment with an equal volume of petroleum jelly (Vaseline) usually overcomes the allergic reaction but naturally the ointment becomes less effective.

Many doubts have been cast on the cosmetic use of vitamin E for the skin. Doctors who use it as a healing agent decry its wholesale, uncontrolled incorporation into cosmetics and feel that the vitamin should be confined to an ointment for medical conditions only. The U.K. authorities have banned advertisement claims for cosmetics containing vitamin E.

INDEX